Vitreoretinal Disorders in Primary Care

Vitreoretinal Disorders
in Primary Care

Thomas H. Williamson

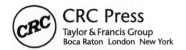

CRC Press
Taylor & Francis Group
Boca Raton London New York

CRC Press is an imprint of the
Taylor & Francis Group, an **informa** business

CRC Press
Taylor & Francis Group
6000 Broken Sound Parkway NW, Suite 300
Boca Raton, FL 33487-2742

International Standard Book Number-13: 978-1-138-62811-3 (Paperback)

Library of Congress Cataloging-in-Publication Data

Names: Williamson, Thomas H., author.
Title: Vitreoretinal disorders in primary care / Thomas H. Williamson.
Description: Boca Raton, FL : CRC Press, [2018] | Includes bibliographical references and index.
Identifiers: LCCN 2017014863| ISBN 9781138096547 (hardback : alk. paper) |
ISBN 9781138628113 (pbk. : alk. paper) | ISBN 9781315210773 (ebook)
Subjects: | MESH: Retinal Diseases--diagnosis | Retinal Diseases--therapy | Vitreous Body | Primary Health Care
Classification: LCC RE551 | NLM WW 270 | DDC 617.7/35--dc23
LC record available at https://lccn.loc.gov/2017014863

Visit the Taylor & Francis Web site at
http://www.taylorandfrancis.com

and the CRC Press Web site at
http://www.crcpress.com

Printed and bound by CPI Group (UK) Ltd, Croydon, CR0 4YY

Contents

Contents

Contents

Preface

The specialism of vitreoretinal surgery has continued to grow in the last 50 years. The main operation of pars plana vitrectomy is now the second most common intraocular operation after cataract surgery. The disorders treated by this surgery are often emergency conditions. The conditions are complex and varied; obtaining or maintaining knowledge of these conditions can be difficult, especially for those in the front line of healthcare provision. This can leave patients vulnerable to error in clinical diagnosis and management. Inappropriate delay in referral can lead to poorer outcomes in these patients.

This book has been written to aid those in the primary care professions to recognise vitreoretinal conditions and provide advice on referral practices. The referral patterns are only a guide, and local practices may vary. It has been assumed for the purposes of the book that there is good access to healthcare facilities and specialist opinion. The recommendations are generalised, and there will be individual patients who require a referral approach different from the one described.

Drawing from my 20 years as an expert witness, I have created fictional medicolegal cases to illustrate how referral may play a part in any potential litigation. These show some of the pitfalls that primary care professionals may experience.

I would like to acknowledge the help of Robin Cannon for the three-dimensional graphics, Professor John Marshall for the histological images of the retina, Dermott Roche for optical coherence tomography images and Matt Robertson for the wide-angle retinal images.

Author

Tom Williamson is a vitreoretinal surgeon located in central London, UK. He has been performing vitreoretinal operations for 30 years and has published widely on the subject. His books are the primary training manuals in vitreoretinal surgery internationally. He has written this book for primary care physicians allowing for informed and safe care of patients with vitreoretinal disorders.

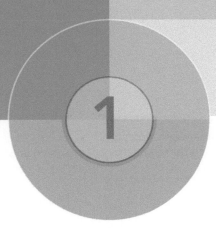

Anatomy and examination of the eye

EMBRYOLOGY OF THE EYE

- 6–7 weeks of gestation:
  The optic cup develops from the optic vesicle and consists of two layers of ectoderm, the outer becoming the retinal pigment epithelium (RPE) and the inner, the neurosensory retina.
- 13 weeks:
  The receptor cells appear.
- 1.5–3 months:
  The RPE becomes pigmented.
- 5.5 months:
  The adult retinal structure can be seen.
- 3–4 months after birth:
  The macula is formed.

ANATOMY

VITREOUS

The vitreous fills the internal space of the eye posterior to the lens and its zonular fibres and has a volume in emmetropia of about 4 mL, which increases to 10 mL in highly myopic eyes. The vitreous is a hypocellular viscous fluid that consists of the following:

- 99% water content
- Hyaluronic acid
- Type 2 collagen fibrils

The cortical part of the vitreous gel has a higher content of hyaluronic acid and collagen compared with the less dense central gel. There are anterior and posterior hyaloid membranes and a central tubular condensation called Cloquet's canal. Removal of the gel does not adversely affect the eye apart from a poorly understood increased risk of nuclear sclerotic cataract.

ANATOMICAL ATTACHMENTS OF THE VITREOUS TO THE SURROUNDING STRUCTURES

- The posterior hyaloid membrane adheres to the internal limiting membrane (ILM) of the retina. This adhesion breaks down in posterior vitreous detachment.
- The vitreous base is a zone of adhesion of the vitreous to the retina and pars plana that is 3–4 mm wide and lying across the ora serrata. It is an area of strong adhesion and is not usually separated even in surgical procedures.
- Weigert's ligament is a circular zone of adhesion of the anterior vitreous, 8–9 mm in diameter, to the posterior lens capsule.
- The posterior hyaloid membrane and the slightly expanded posterior limit of Cloquet's canal meet around the margin of the optic disc. During posterior vitreous detachment, evidence of this adhesion is seen as Weiss's ring.
- A circle of relatively increased adhesion to the retina may be present in the parafoveal area and implicated in macular hole formation (Figures 1.1 and 1.2).

RETINA

The retina is divided into regions.

- The macula between the temporal vascular arcades serves approximately 20° of visual field.
- The fovea is a central darkened area with a pit called the foveola.

The cones, the receptors for detailed vision, are densest at the fovea, at 15,000/mm^2, with 4,000–5,000/mm^2 in the macula. There are 6 million cones and 120 million rods in total (Figure 1.3).

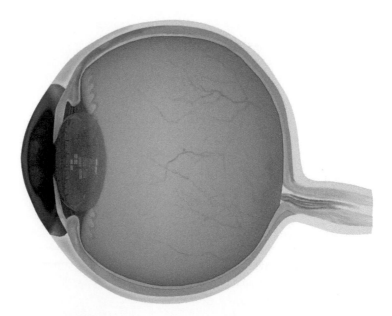

Figure 1.1 Cutaway of the eye showing the vitreous cavity filled with vitreous gel.

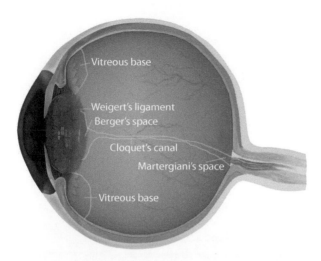

Figure 1.2 Vitreous anatomy is shown.

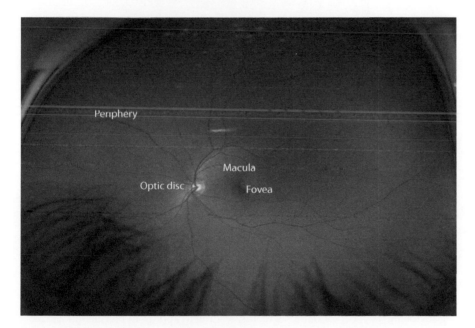

Figure 1.3 Landmarks of the normal retina are shown.

The retina is organised into four layers of cells and two layers of neuronal connections. It has a structural cell called the Muller cell, which extends through all the layers. These are as follows:

- Specialised glial cells
- A sink of ions during depolarisation of receptors
- Layer involved in cone neuroprotection
- Layer controlling vascular permeability and haemostasis
- Layer involved in pigment recycling

There are astrocytes and microglial cells in addition in the retina (Figure 1.4).

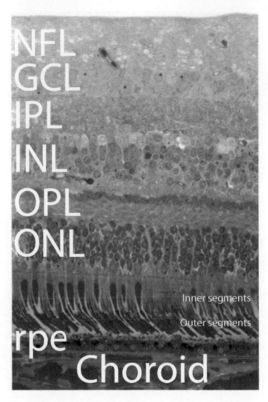

Figure 1.4 Anatomical layers of the retina are shown. GCL, ganglion cell layer; IPL, inner plexiform layer; INL, inner nuclear layer; NFL, nerve fibre layer; OPL, outer plexiform layer; ONL, outer nuclear layer.

RETINAL PIGMENT EPITHELIUM

The RPE is a single layer of pigmented cuboidal epithelial cells, which look after the function of the receptors by performing the following:

- Absorbing stray light (using melanin pigment)
- Transporting metabolites between the receptors and the choroid
- Providing a blood retinal barrier
- Regenerating the visual pigments
- Phagocytosing the receptor outer segments, leading to lipofuscin production

PHOTORECEPTOR LAYER

The photoreceptor transduces light into neuronal signals. The action of light closes gated cation channels leading to hyperpolarisation of the cell. Two types of photoreceptor exist, the rods predominantly in the periphery and absent from the fovea and the cones concentrated at the macula.

The receptors consist of two parts:

- Outer segments
    Light is absorbed by the visual pigments in stacked discs, separate in the rods (1,000 in number), interconnected in the cones. This is joined to the inner segment by the cilium.

- Inner segments

  These consist of an inner myoid, which contains the Golgi apparatus and ribosomes for making cell structures, and an outer ellipsoid, which contains mitochondria for energy production. These connect to the nucleus by the outer connecting fibre. The inner connecting fibre connects to the synaptic region. The latter has synapses arranged as triads with connections to one bipolar cell and two horizontal cells. In cones, there may be up to 20 triads, whereas the rods have only one.

CONES

Cones provide high-resolution colour vision in photopic conditions. They react quickly and recover rapidly to different light stimuli. Three types of cone photoreceptor exist in the human eye with different opsin proteins bound to a common chromophore (11-*cis*-retinal). The three types provide sensitivities which peak at different light wavelengths with short S cones at 420 nm (blue), middle M cones at 530 nm (green) and long L cones at 560 nm (red) (Figure 1.5).

- Outer limiting layer

  This consists of junctional complexes from the Muller cells and photoreceptors and is located at the inner connecting fibres.
- Outer plexiform layer

  The cell processes of the horizontal cells and bipolar cells synapse with the receptors.
- Intermediary neurons
- Inner nuclear layer

  This contains the cell bodies of the bipolar cells, Muller cells, amacrine cells and horizontal cells.
- Inner plexiform layer

  The bipolar cells axons pass through, synapsing with the amacrine cells, which help process the neuronal signals to the ganglion cells.

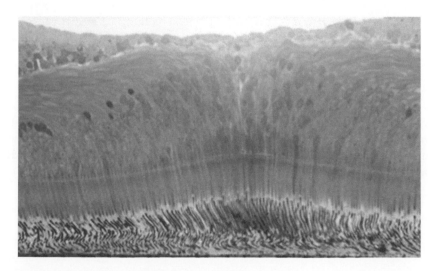

Figure 1.5 Fovea has a high density of cones.

GANGLION CELLS

- Ganglion cell layer
  The cell bodies of the ganglion cells are found here. These cells have gathered preprocessed information from the other retinal cells. At the macula, there is one ganglion cell to one receptor, but on average in the whole retina, there is one for 130 receptors.

NERVE FIBRE LAYER

The nerve fibres of the ganglion cells on the inner surface of the retina pass tangentially towards the optic nerve.

INNER LIMITING MEMBRANE

The ILM is a tough membrane laid down by the Muller cells with connections to the hyaloid membrane of the vitreous.

RETINAL BLOOD VESSELS

The central retinal artery supplies the neural retina with the exception of the photoreceptors, which are supplied by the choriocapillaris. The former is an end artery system with a single draining vessel, the central retinal vein. Both the central retinal artery and the vein have four main branches, which divide at the optic disc to supply nasal and temporal quadrants. At the posterior pole, there is a capillary network at the level of the nerve fibre layer and the outer plexiform layer. In the periphery, there is one capillary network at the inner nuclear layer. The capillary endothelium forms the inner retinal blood retinal barrier by having tight intercellular junctions (Figure 1.6).

BRUCH'S MEMBRANE

Bruch's membrane is a pentilaminar structure partly representing the basement membranes of the RPE and the choriocapillaris. It is of ectodermal and mesodermal origins. The accumulation of damage in Bruch's membrane is seen in age-related macular degeneration.

CHOROID

This is a vascular layer (large vessels are outer and the capillaries are inner) with a highly relative blood flow and low oxygen utilisation (3%). It supplies the RPE and photoreceptors. The highly anastomotic and fenestrated capillaries are arranged into lobules and are supplied by the posterior ciliary arteries and drained by the vortex veins.

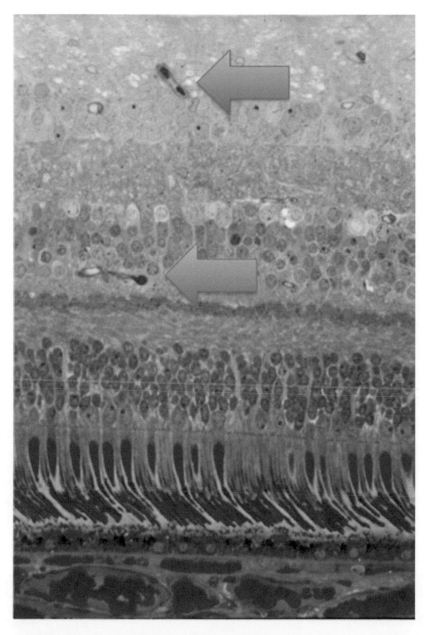

Figure 1.6 At the posterior pole, there is a capillary network at the level of the nerve fibre layer and the outer plexiform layer. In the periphery, there is one capillary network at the inner nuclear layer. The capillary endothelium forms the inner retinal blood retina barrier by having tight intercellular junctions.

INVESTIGATION

VISUAL ACUITY

LogMar values are recommended for the ease of analysis of data for surgical audit and governance. This can be measured by the Snellen chart or Early Treatment Diabetic Retinopathy Study chart but requires full refractive correction.

SLIT LAMP

Goldman tonometry, various contact lenses or three-mirror contact lenses can be used. The operator can visualise the vitreous by looking behind the posterior lens. The slit lamp allows the use of specialised lenses for the examination of the retina, e.g. super-field 90D or 60D non-contact lenses.

OPTICAL COHERENCE TOMOGRAPHY

Optical coherence tomography (OCT), first developed for ophthalmic imaging in the 1990s[1] is invaluable in the retinal clinic. OCT scanning provides two-dimensional cross sections of the retina from which three-dimensional reconstructions can be created.[2] Conceptually, OCT operates on the same physical principles as an ultrasound scan except it uses light as the carrier signal. The spatial resolution of an OCT is conventionally 10–20 MHz.

The source of light in an OCT is produced by a superluminescent diode, a femtosecond laser, or more recently using white light.[3]

OCT works by splitting a beam of light into two arms – a reference arm and a sampling arm.

First-generation OCTs are time-domain OCT, so named because the length of the reference arm is varied with time, in order to correlate with the back-reflected sample arm. This is achieved with the use of an adjustable mirror of known distance within the device. The sample arm is focused onto the retina with the use of an in-built 78D lens. The sample beam is reflected off the structures in the eye and is recombined with the reference beam by using a Michelson interferometer within the unit. A single cycle of this process yields one A-scan. This single scan is composed of data on the distance the sample arm has travelled and the back reflectance and backscatter of the beam. Tissue layers at varying depths and optical characteristics produce differing reflective intensities (Figure 1.7).

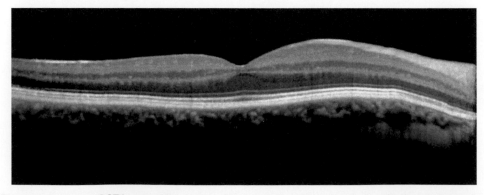

Figure 1.7 Normal OCT image of the macula. The foveal dip is shown centrally, with the nasal macular retina on the right.

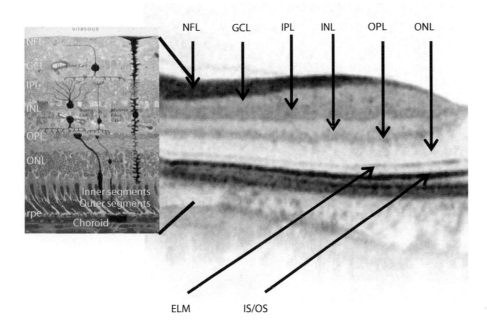

Figure 1.8 Various layers of the retina are shown on OCT. The IS/OS border also named the ellipsoid layer is a good indicator of the health of the retinal receptors. ELM, external limiting membrane; GCL, ganglion cell layer; IPL, inner plexiform layer; INL, inner nuclear layer; NFL, nerve fibre layer; OPL, outer plexiform layer; ONL, outer nuclear layer.

As in an ultrasound scan, in order to produce a B-scan image, multiple A-scans are obtained in rapid succession across the area of interest. Software combines this information to produce a two-dimensional image either in greyscale or with arbitrary false colouring. The result is a cross-sectional scan; a reconstructed three-dimensional topographical image, with quantitative thickness measurements; or more recently, z-plane or coronal scans.[3]

- The inner retina has moderate reflectance.
- Receptors have low reflectance.
- RPE shows high scatter from melanin.

The laser is thereafter blocked, and less information from the choroid is usually obtained. Measurements of the tissues in the z-axis are possible to quantify retinal thickness and volume (Figure 1.8).

INNER SEGMENT AND OUTER SEGMENT JUNCTION (ELLIPSOID LAYER)

This is the band correlating to the junction of the inner and outer segment (IS/OS) of the photoreceptors. The IS/OS band is a high-reflectance signal at this junction resulting from the abrupt change in the refractive index stemming from the highly organised stacks of membranous discs in the photoreceptor outer segment.[4] Visual acuity has been significantly correlated with OCT detection of the IS/OS junction in the following:

- Retinitis pigmentosa[5]
- Macula-off retinal detachments[6]
- Full-thickness macular holes[7-9]
- Central serous chorioretinopathy[10]
- Age-related macular degeneration[11]
- Macular oedema associated with branch retinal vein occlusions[12,13]

CENTRAL RETINAL THICKNESS

The central retinal thickness (CRT) is the simplest measure to use and has been quoted in numerous studies. CRT was compared between six commercially available OCT scanners in a study involving healthy eyes, and a variation of between 0.45% and 3.33% was found. The slightly different segmentation algorithms employed by each device explained the discrepancies.[14] In effect, this means that the line that the software uses to determine the outer retinal boundary differs, and so different OCT systems should not be used interchangeably.

SUBJECTIVE TESTS

The retinal patient often complains of symptoms, which are related to the dysfunction of the macula such as distortion and change in image size.

At present the methods available to assess these are limited. Amsler charts can be used at the most basic level to determine distortion.

REFERENCES

1. Huang, D., Swanson, E. A., Lin, C. P. et al. Optical coherence tomography. *Science* 1991;254(5035):1178–81.
2. Hee, M. R., Izatt, J. A., Swanson, E. A. et al. Optical coherence tomography of the human retina. *Arch Ophthalmol* 1995;113(3):325–32.
3. Sacchet, D., Moreau, J., Georges, P. and Dubois A. Simultaneous dual-band ultra-high resolution full-field optical coherence tomography. *Opt Express* 2008;16(24):19434–46.
4. Chan, A., Duker, J. S., Ishikawa, H. et al. Quantification of photoreceptor layer thickness in normal eyes using optical coherence tomography. *Retina* 2006;26(6):655–60.
5. Aizawa, S., Mitamura, Y., Baba, T. et al. Correlation between visual function and photoreceptor inner/outer segment junction in patients with retinitis pigmentosa. *Eye* 2009;23(2):304–8.
6. Wakabayashi, T., Oshima, Y., Fujimoto, H. et al. Foveal microstructure and visual acuity after retinal detachment repair: Imaging analysis by Fourier-domain optical coherence tomography. *Ophthalmology* 2009;116(3):519–28.
7. Sano, M., Shimoda, Y., Hashimoto, H. and Kishi, S. Restored photoreceptor outer segment and visual recovery after macular hole closure. *Am J Ophthalmol* 2009;147(2):313–8 e1.
8. Baba, T., Yamamoto, S., Arai, M. et al. Correlation of visual recovery and presence of photoreceptor inner/outer segment junction in optical coherence images after successful macular hole repair. *Retina* 2008;28(3):453–8.

9. Inoue, M., Watanabe, Y., Arakawa, A. et al. Spectral-domain optical coherence tomography images of inner/outer segment junctions and macular hole surgery outcomes. *Graefes Arch Clin Exp Ophthalmol* 2009;247(3):325–30.

10. Piccolino, F. C., de la Longrais, R. R., Ravera, G. et al. The foveal photoreceptor layer and visual acuity loss in central serous chorioretinopathy. *Am J Ophthalmol* 2005;139(1):87–99.

11. Sayanagi, K., Sharma, S., Yamamoto, T. and Kaiser, P. K. Comparison of spectral-domain versus time-domain optical coherence tomography in management of age-related macular degeneration with ranibizumab. *Ophthalmology* 2009;116(5):947–55.

12. Ota, M., Tsujikawa, A., Murakami, T. et al. Foveal photoreceptor layer in eyes with persistent cystoid macular edema associated with branch retinal vein occlusion. *Am J Ophthalmol* 2008;145(2):273–80.

13. Murakami, T., Tsujikawa, A., Ohta, M. et al. Photoreceptor status after resolved macular edema in branch retinal vein occlusion treated with tissue plasminogen activator. *Am J Ophthalmol* 2007;143(1):171–3.

14. Wolf-Schnurrbusch, U. E., Ceklic, L., Brinkmann, C. K. et al. Macular thickness measurements in healthy eyes using six different optical coherence tomography instruments. *Invest Ophthalmol Vis Sci* 2009;50(7):3432–7.

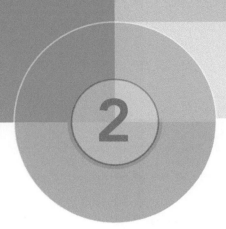

Posterior vitreous detachment

2

INTRODUCTION

Posterior vitreous detachment (PVD) is the most common and most important event that occurs in the vitreous. As the vitreous ages, the normal architectural features degrade causing the following:

- Syneresis
- Lacuna (cavity) formation
- Collapse of the vitreous gel

The collagen disintegrates and aggregates, giving rise to *floaters*.[1,2] Pathologically, there is a loss of sodium hyaluronate[3] and an increase in vitreous mobility with age[4] (Figure 2.1).

Most individuals will develop PVD (separation of the posterior hyaloid membrane from the internal limiting membrane), without symptoms, or pathological consequences, usually between the ages of 40 and 80 years:

- Twenty-seven per cent of patients in their seventh decade have PVD.
- Sixty-three per cent of patients in their eighth decade have PVD.[5]

This may occur very occasionally at a younger age (less than 40 years old) in myopia, diabetes, retinal vascular disorders, trauma and retinitis pigmentosa.[6–11] Presentation with symptomatic PVD (flashes and floaters) may be more common in females than in males and in myopia[12]; however, more retinal tears occur in males.[13]

The detached posterior hyaloid membrane becomes wrinkled and usually separates completely from the retina up to the posterior border of the vitreous base. It will remain attached to the vitreoretinal adhesions such as lattice degeneration or chorioretinal scars.

- No racial differences in the rates of PVD have been found between white and Asian races.
- It is suspected that black races have less PVD.[14–16]
- The fellow eye shows evidence of PVD in 90% in 3 years.[17]
- Eleven per cent develop symptomatic PVD in the other eye in 2 years.[18]

PVD causes most rhegmatogenous retinal detachments (RRDs) via retinal tear formation. It is the instigator of the disorders of macular pucker and macular hole formation. PVD may tear blood vessels in the retina or in neovascular complexes causing haemorrhaging into the vitreous cavity.

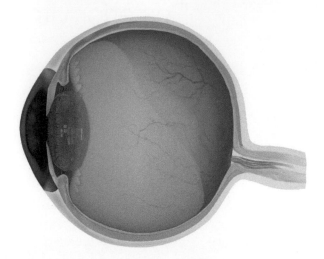

Figure 2.1 Vitreous may separate away from the retina in PVD.

Table 2.1 Vitreoretinal conditions and the vitreous

Caused by age-related PVD	Retinal breaks
	RRD
	Macular epiretinal membrane (ERM) and vitreomacular traction syndrome
	Macular hole
	Vitreous haemorrhage
Associated with pathological vitreous separation	Diabetic tractional retinal detachment
	Complications of posterior uveitis
	Trauma

Acute ischaemic events such as retinal vein occlusion may induce PVD with an increased prevalence of PVD 1 year after the onset of the vein occlusion.[19]

The importance of PVD has led to methods for the inducement of PVD[20–27] such as plasmin injection as a proteolytic acting on the vitreoretinal interface and has recently been commercialised as ocriplasmin injections.[28]

The most reliable clinical sign of PVD is a ring of tissue on the posterior vitreous surface, in front of the optic disc (Weiss's ring). The ring is often incomplete and is absent in 13%[29,30] of PVD.

Patients describe a 'cobweb' or 'spider' or 'fly' which moves with eye movements. OCT has revealed that many adults have an incomplete PVD not visible on biomicroscopy but with separation of the posterior hyaloid membrane from the retina with residual attachments at the optic disc or the fovea (Table 2.1).[31]

SYMPTOMS

FLOATERS

Floaters must be discriminated from paracentral scotomata. Ask the patient to describe the floater that should have momentum as the eye moves, i.e. the floater will move with the eye but will continue to move when the eye stops before finally returning to its original position and resting there. In contrast, a scotoma remains in the same position (relative to fixation) in all

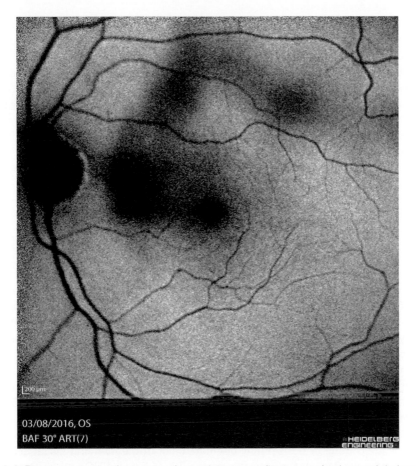

Figure 2.2 Floater caused by vitreous opacity can be seen easily on scanning laser ophthalmoscopy.

positions of gaze. The patient may also describe the floater as something in front of the vision or 'in the way' of the vision, whereas most scotoma are negative (the vision is missing in the area of scotoma), although some may be positive (e.g. the zigzags of a migraine).

Floaters can be characterised by multiple presentations, e.g. cobwebs, veils, rings, a single spot or multiple spots. These come from the thickened posterior hyaloid membrane, Weiss ring or cells that have been dispersed into the vitreous (cells are seen by the patient as small round spots). Floaters that occur before the age of 40 years and are chronic in presentation are most often due to vitreous degeneration without PVD (vitreous syneresis). However, it may only take a single floater of recent onset to indicate the development of a PVD (Figure 2.2).

FLASHES

Introduction

Photopsia is the experience of light from non-photic stimulation.

- The first description was from Purkinje in 1819,[32] who attributed them to traction on the retina.
- In 1935, Moore[33] described them as 'lightning streaks' with a 'flash-like appearance of the lights; their position, sometimes slanting but usually vertical and almost always

to the outer side of the eyes, persisting for periods of up to three months; and their association with the sudden development of muscae volitantes or the presence of visible vitreous opacities'.

- In 1940, he described more cases and called them lightning flashes.[34] He developed streaks in his own eye in 1947.[35] He initially thought the phenomenon to be innocent but commented in his paper that 'I used systematically to dilate the pupils and to take the visual fields in fear lest they might indicate some early organic retinal lesion, such as a commencing detachment, vascular disease, or perhaps an early neoplasm'.[33]
- The photopsia were correctly attributed to PVD by Verhoeff[36] in 1941.
- The risk of retinal detachment associated with lightning flashes was discovered by Berens et al.[37] in 1954.
- In 2008, rare 'black flashes' were described at the commencement of the PVD[38] and attributed to traction of the vitreous on the optic nerve head.

Clinical characteristics

Patients usually have 'lightning flashes' in the temporal periphery of their visual field that last a second or so. Their exact pathogenesis is obscure but may be due to depolarisation of the receptors from tugging of the vitreous base on the retina or by impact of the vitreous on the peripheral retina. The patient may describe that the flashes occur on eye movements. After repeated eye movements over a short time, the flashes gradually reduce in severity. The flashes are better seen in the dark.

In a very few patients, black temporal flashes are experienced by the patient for a few hours before the lightning flashes and floaters occur[38] possibly produced by the Weiss ring pulling on the optic nerve head before it separates. This may indicate a block of axoplasmic flow in the superficial nerve fibres.

Typically, the lightning flashes of PVD are vertical, temporally placed and instantaneous.[39] If the flashes are oblique or horizontally orientated, not in the temporal visual field or not typical instantaneous flashes, the patient is more likely to have a PVD with a retinal tear or RRD.[39]

Flashes occur with many other disorders, such as the zigzag lights of migraine, flickering stars associated with occipital ischaemia and rarely cultured lights of the acute zonal outer occult retinopathy syndromes. Mostly, these photopsia are centrally placed in the visual field and, therefore, easy to discriminate from those from PVD. Slower peripheral flashes are produced by the leading edge of some retinal detachments often shaped like a comet's tail.

Patients who experience symptoms during posterior vitreous separation have a 10% risk of developing a retinal tear.[40–42]

Flashes from PVD usually subside in a few months while floaters get less.[43] The floaters lessen not only because the opacities on the posterior surface of the vitreous sink lower in the eye, but also because they move anteriorly further away from the retina.

Severe floaters can be bothersome, and a few patients will require a pars plana vitrectomy (PPV) to clear the vision. It is however prudent to wait to see if the symptoms subside before a referral for consideration for surgical intervention is given.

Rarely, flashes will persist for years usually associated with vitreous-attached RRD in a young myope (i.e. flashes associated with RRD rather than PVD) and very rarely after PVD. Occasionally, patients will have flashes after vitrectomy surgery, illustrating that we are unsure of their source (Table 2.2).

Table 2.2 Different presentations of flashes

Diagnosis	Duration	Colour	Location	Shape	Stimulus	Other symptoms	Flickering
PVD	Seconds or less	White	Temporal periphery	Crescentic vertical	Eye movements	Floaters	No
Migraine	20–30 minutes	Not typically	Paracentral	Arcuate, zigzag	Stress, food	Scotoma, headache, nausea	Yes
Occipital ischaemia	Minutes	Nil	Central	Petaloid	Neck movements, exertion		Yes
Cystoid macular oedema	Constant	Variable	Central	Pinpricks	Nil	Poor vision	Yes
Outer retinal or RPE abnormality	Minutes	Blue/purple	Paracentral	Blobs, spirals	Nil	Scotoma	No
Retinal detachment	Seconds	Golden	Central/ paracentral	Comet oblique horizontal	Eye movements	Visual field loss	No

SIGNS

DETECTION OF PVD

A PVD can be diagnosed by examining the eye with a 90-dioptre lens. If a Weiss ring is present, then a PVD has occurred. The posterior hyaloid membrane may be seen. A partial PVD is a diagnosis that should be made only rarely because it can be extremely difficult to determine whether there are remaining vitreous attachments. Attachments at the optic disc, chorioretinal scars and epiretinal membranes at the macula and neovascular tissue may be seen. Usually, a PVD occurs completely, soon after the onset of symptoms (within a few hours). In only a few patients will the PVD progress over a few weeks. These patients may show new retinal breaks with tears seen at 6 weeks after the onset of symptoms in 1.8–3.4%[44] (Figures 2.3 and 2.4).

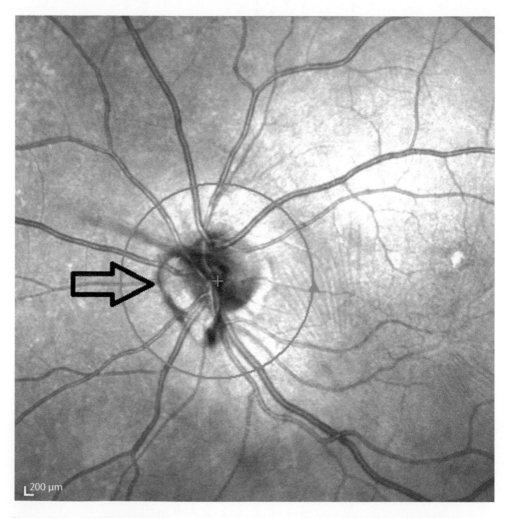

Figure 2.3 Weiss ring can be seen in front of the optic nerve of this eye (there is some epiretinal membrane [ERM] in addition).

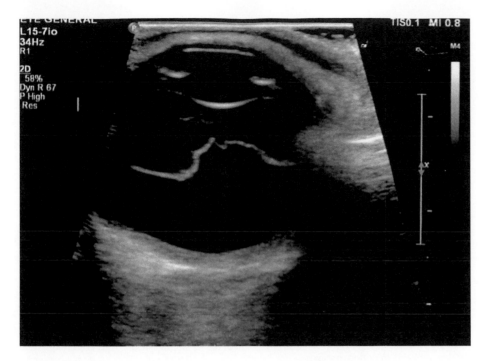

Figure 2.4 Posterior surface of the vitreous can be seen on this ultrasound.

SHAFER'S SIGN

In most patients with retinal tears, retinal pigment epithelial cells, which migrate from the subretinal space through the tear, will be visible in the anterior vitreous (Shafer's sign). This is highly predictive of a retinal tear with approximately 90% with the sign having a retinal tear and only 10% without the sign having a tear.[41,45–48]

The pigment granules in Shafer's sign are relatively large (diameter of 30–50 μm), brown (coffee-coloured) and are seen in the anterior vitreous. The patient, therefore, should be examined during up and down eye movements allowing the inferior vitreous to present itself for examination in the pupil. Only one granule is required to make the diagnosis of Shafer's sign, indicating a risk of a retinal tear (Figure 2.5).

VITREOUS HAEMORRHAGE

Red blood cells (RBCs), which are smaller in size (6–8 μm), may also be seen and should raise suspicion of pathology, although this is less indicative than pigment granules (50% of patients with RBCs in vitreous having retinal tears). Sometimes the haemorrhage is severe, preventing the visualisation of all or part of the retina. This should be investigated by ultrasound and a referral for a PPV performed urgently to allow detection of breaks. In some patients, a superior break might be seen, but the inferior retina is obscured by haemorrhage. The surgeon may laser the superior break and observe. However, it may be safer to proceed to PPV because of the chance of multiple breaks (approximately 50–60%), which might be missed in the obscured retina (Figure 2.6).

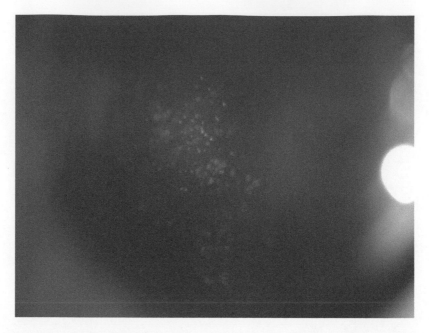

Figure 2.5 Pigment granules in the vitreous are a sign of retinal tear formation. They are often described as looking like coffee granules.

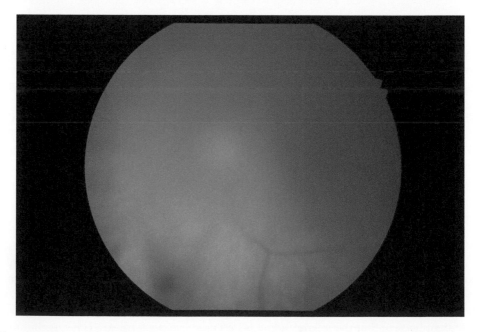

Figure 2.6 View of the retina is obscured by a vitreous haemorrhage.

Table 2.3 Other signs of PVD

Sign	Odds ratio for detection of a retinal break	95% Confidence interval
Subjective vision reduction	5.0	3.1–8.1
Vitreous haemorrhage	10	5.1–20
Absence of vitreous pigmentation	0.23	0.12–0.43

Source: Hollands, H. et al., *JAMA*, 302, 2243–9, 2009.

OPHTHALMOSCOPY

Note that the patient requires 360° examination of the retina with indirect ophthalmoscopy. The indentation of the far periphery is the gold-standard examination. This aids in the identification of breaks both by introducing peripheral retina into the view and allowing a dynamic examination of a break. The break can be opened up and more clearly seen by the movement of the retina over the indented sclera. Moving the choroid under the break changes the colour of the choroid seen through the break. Retinal haemorrhage and pigmentation both remain the same colour despite indentation.

If a patient presents early with PVD, re-examine the retina at 6 weeks after the symptoms have started because 1.8–3.4% will have new tears seen at the second examination.[49] If patients have vitreous haemorrhage, retinal haemorrhage or develop new symptoms in the intervening period, they may be more likely to have breaks seen at the second examination.

Note that if a patient presents very early with PVD symptoms after a few days, another examination at 1–2 weeks is useful in the case that the vitreous has not yet fully separated (Table 2.3).

PVD may induce haemorrhages of the optic disc (sometimes causing subtle visual field loss)[50,51] or peripheral or macular retinal haemorrhages.[52,53]

RETINAL TEARS

U TEARS

In PVD with symptoms, 10% of patients will develop retinal tears. Most tears are found at the first visit. Ten per cent of tears are reportedly detected at 6 weeks from onset of symptoms (constituting theoretically 1% of all cases with symptomatic PVD).[46,54,55] Breaks found in asymptomatic eyes with PVD are less likely to lead to retinal detachment[56] probably because the tear has been present for a while and has not progressed.

U tears (or other tears caused by PVD) require treatment by either laser retinopexy or cryotherapy. U tears present with the base of their flaps anteriorly in the direction of the traction of the vitreous. The aim of retinopexy should be to surround the whole tear. Tears close to the ora serrata can be treated by retinopexy around the tear and up to the ora serrata. Retinopexy should be performed soon after the diagnosis, e.g. the same day. Retinopexy should be secured after 2 weeks, preventing progression to retinal detachment (Figure 2.7).

Posteriorly placed holes can be treated with laser therapy employing a contact lens or a super-field lens. More anterior tears may require indirect laser ophthalmoscopy and indentation. Alternatively, cryotherapy retinopexy can be applied with a local anaesthetic injection in the conjunctiva of the eye. These are specialist skills, and therefore, referral is required (Figures 2.8 and 2.9).

Note that retinal tears are often multiple (50–60% of the eyes).

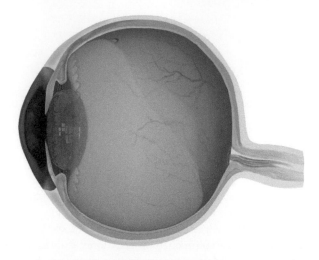

Figure 2.7 PVD may tear the retina through traction on the retina creating a retinal break (hole).

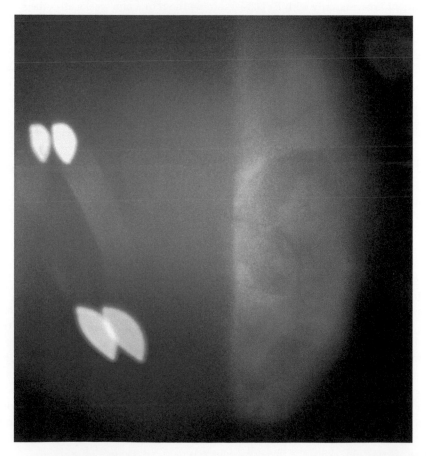

Figure 2.8 U tear with a bridging vessel and a tear inferior to it seen with slit lamp and superfield lens.

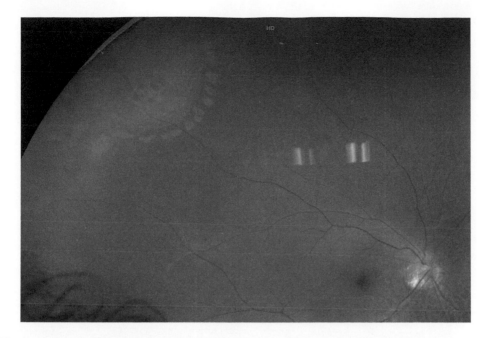

Figure 2.9 Retinal break with minimal fluid treated first with laser and then with cryotherapy.

ATROPHIC ROUND HOLES

Flat round holes are often seen in asymptomatic myopic eyes associated with snail track or lattice degeneration and often in patients who are 20–40 years old. The vitreous is attached. In most circumstances, these holes do not need to be treated.

Retinal detachment associated with round holes in an asymptomatic eye is unlikely to be progressive to retinal detachment with an approximate risk of 1:200.[57,58] Round hole-related retinal detachments can progress to the fovea but usually slowly.[59] A retinal surgeon who will discuss whether surgery is required should assess them. The patient should be made aware of the small risk and the symptomatology of retinal detachment progressing (Figure 2.10).

OTHER BREAKS

Paravascular tears are associated with paravascular lattice degeneration (seen in Stickler's syndrome). These tears should be treated immediately. Other breaks such as retinal dialysis and giant retinal tears usually present with retinal detachment and are therefore not amenable to prophylaxis and need surgery.

PROGRESSION TO RETINAL DETACHMENT

Any subretinal fluid around the hole indicates that fluid has entered under the retina from the vitreous cavity, and there is now a retinal detachment present. A surgical procedure is usually required (see future chapters).

Figure 2.10 Round retinal hole.

PERIPHERAL RETINAL DEGENERATIONS

A number of peripheral degenerations will be seen in the retina.

- Associated with retinal break formation
    1. Lattice degeneration is an equatorial, circumferential hyalinisation of the retinal blood vessels with associated pigmentation giving a criss-crossed pattern. It is often associated with round retinal holes and can be associated with U-shaped tears if a PVD has occurred. It is present in 5% of eyes but more frequently in moderate myopia.[60,61] Long-term studies suggest that the chance of tractional tears is 2.9% in 10 years, but the risk of retinal detachment remains low.[62] For this reason, routine treatment of lattice with laser retinopexy has largely been abandoned. In addition, many holes that occur with retinal detachment appear out with the areas of lattice[63]; therefore, treating the lattice areas does not prevent tear formation. The radial lattice in a paravascular orientation may indicate risk of slit-like paravascular tears. Stickler's syndrome should be suspected (Figure 2.11).
    2. Snail track degeneration has no pigmentation and is associated with round tears and retinal detachment with attached vitreous gel. More often seen in the black population, it is probably a variant of lattice degeneration (Figure 2.12).[64]

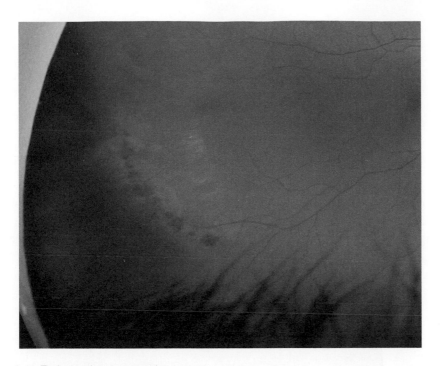

Figure 2.11 Typical lattice degeneration.

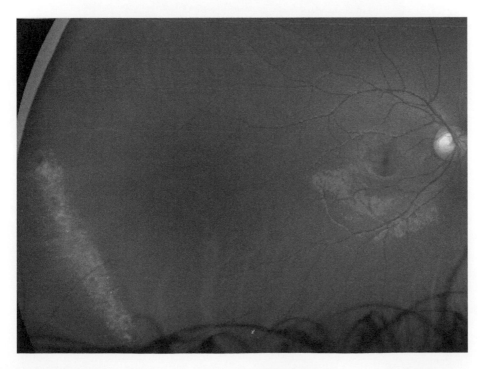

Figure 2.12 Snail track peripheral degeneration can be associated with round retinal holes.

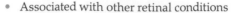

- Associated with other retinal conditions
  3. Reticular degeneration is a honeycombed pigmentary change occurring in the aged population. It is associated with age-related macular degeneration (Figure 2.13).[65,66]
  4. Microcystic changes may be seen as tiny yellow flecks, and this can be associated with retinoschisis formation (Figures 2.14 and 2.15).
- Others
  5. Cobblestone degeneration is characterised by punched-out atrophic areas of depigmentation of the choroid and retina (Figure 2.16).
  6. White without pressure shows a crenated edge with the pallor of the retina, more obvious in highly pigmented fundi. There is a vague association with giant retinal tear formation (Figure 2.17).
  7. Ora serrata changes such as oral cysts, bays and meridional complexes may also be seen. Studies on prophylaxis in retinal detachment do not meet the standards of statistical scrutiny,[64] but retinopexy of these lesions is generally thought to be not required.

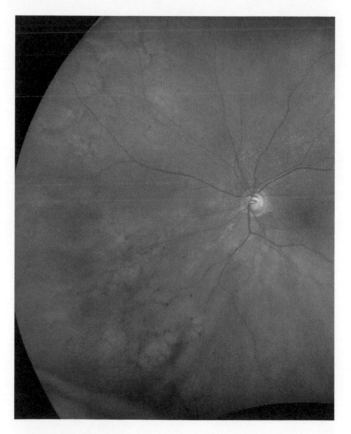

Figure 2.13 Reticular degeneration of the retinal periphery.

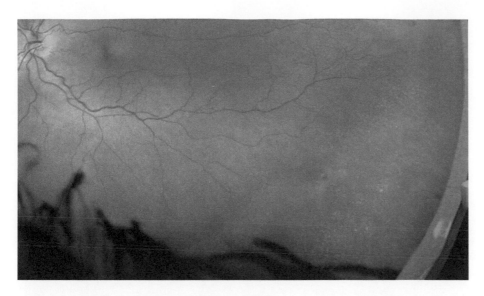

Figure 2.14 Microcytic changes in the periphery of the eye.

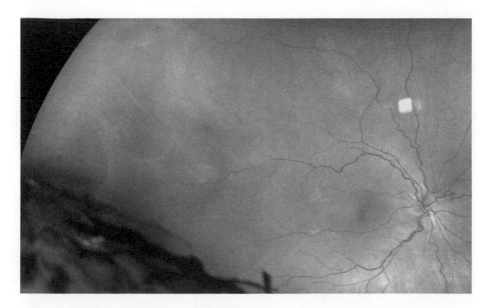

Figure 2.15 Outer leaf breaks from retinoschisis in the other eye of the patient with microcytic changes.

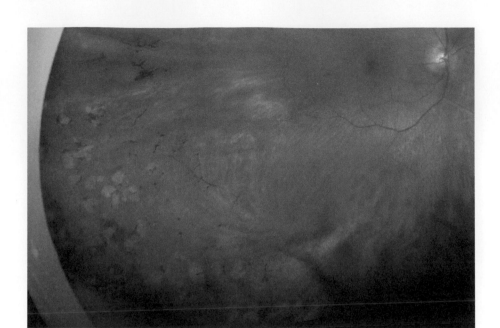

Figure 2.16 Cobblestone degeneration in the retinal periphery.

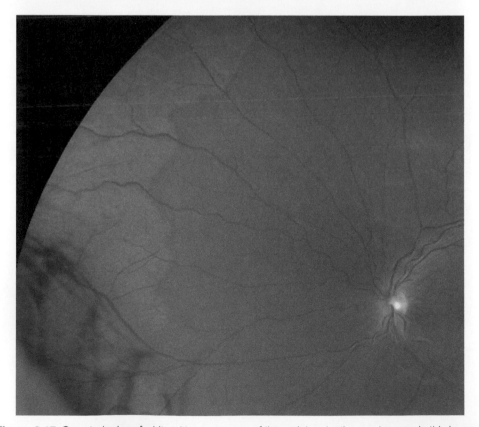

Figure 2.17 Crenated edge of white without pressure of the peripheral retina can be seen in this image.

REFERRAL

POSTERIOR VITREOUS DETACHMENT

Correct referral of PVD requires the identification of the following:

- At-risk population: over 40 years old
- Correct symptoms: discriminate floaters from scotomata
- Correct description of photopsia

The confidence and ability of the referring physician to thoroughly examine the vitreous for Shaffer's sign and the retina for retinal breaks determines the referral practice required. If there is no ability to do these tasks, then immediate referral for review within 24 hours is recommended. Some may be able to examine the vitreous for pigment cells and, if negative, have more confidence that there is no retinal break. In which case, referral can be made over a slightly longer time scale if desired. Others will be able to examine the retina with some confidence; however, the gold-standard retinal examination to categorically exclude retinal tears would be with binocular indirect ophthalmoscopy and indentation or slit lamp examination with three-mirror lens application. These tend to be specialist skills not available in primary care. Therefore, a referral is required.

The highest risk period is with symptoms of less than a 6-week duration. Within that period, the referral should be immediate (<24 hours). The risk of a retinal tear, which will lead to retinal detachment, appears to be much less after the 6-week duration of symptoms, in which case, the referral can be less urgent and the patient can be seen in weeks rather than days (Table 2.4).

If retinal breaks are seen, the patient should be referred on the same day for treatment before RRD occurs.

Retinal breaks associated with PVD will not always lead to RRD (50% are thought to detach). Some retinal breaks that have remained flat will therefore be occasionally seen during routine examination in an asymptomatic patient. These will often have pigmented margins. They do not need treatment, but if in doubt, refer for review.

Operculated retinal breaks where the break flap has pulled off the retina and can be seen on the vitreous are believed to have less risk of progression to retinal detachment. However, the information available on this is scanty, and these tears are best referred on urgently.

Round retinal breaks in asymptomatic eyes with an attached retina can be detected routinely on review. These are no longer treated prophylactically as they are regarded as low risk, 1:200, for progression to RRD.

Similarly, peripheral degenerations such as lattice, although associated with an increased risk of RRD, are no longer treated with prophylactic retinopexy because the risk rate is thought to be low.

Table 2.4 Symptomatic PVD

Condition	Characteristics	Referral	Why?
Symptomatic PVD	Symptoms less than 6 weeks	Immediate	Risk of retinal breaks
	Symptoms more than 6 weeks	Routine	Risk of retinal breaks leading to RRD is low

MISSING THE SYMPTOMS OF POSTERIOR VITREOUS DETACHMENT

A patient goes to see his family medical practitioner (FP) with 1 month of flashes and floaters in one eye and some blurring of vision. The patient is advised to go to an optician for a dilated eye examination. The optician records good vision and, after dilation of the pupils, finds no problems with the retina.

ERROR

The optician misses a retinal break (or Shafer's sign) but attempts to examine the eye appropriately in a primary care setting.

The patient then attends another FP 1 week later and again describes flashes and floaters and reduced vision. The FP does not check the patient's vision or dilate the eyes. The FP refers to the hospital by letter, but there is a delay in the preparation of the letter.

ERRORS

No visual acuity check means the macula may or may not have been detached. The referral process is too slow by letter.

The patient suffers a further reduction in vision and attends a local hospital. A macula-off retinal detachment with a retinal tear is found. Surgery is performed and the retina is reattached with good visual acuity recovery.

Luckily, the patient notices his vision getting worse and attends ophthalmology, allowing RRD diagnosis and treatment, restricting further delay and allowing good visual acuity recovery.

The patient has good visual acuity but complains of a difference in the size of the images in the eyes. The operated eye sees a smaller image and some distortion.

The postoperative symptoms are related to the macula off retinal detachment, which could have been avoided if the optician and FPs had recognized the risks and referred more promptly.

The patient can sue for the delay in diagnosis and referral and the subsequent loss of vision and persistent symptoms.

REFERENCES

1. Bishop, P. N., Holmes, D. F., Kadler, K. E. et al. Age-related changes on the surface of vitreous collagen fibrils. *Invest Ophthalmol Vis Sci* 2004;45(4):1041–6.
2. Akiba, J., Ueno, N. and Chakrabarti B. Molecular mechanisms of posterior vitreous detachment. *Graefes Arch Clin Exp Ophthalmol* 1993;231(7):408–12.
3. Larsson, L. and Osterlin, S. Posterior vitreous detachment: A combined clinical and physiochemical study. *Graefes Arch Clin Exp Ophthalmol* 1985;223(2):92–5.
4. Walton, K. A., Meyer, C. H., Harkrider, C. J. et al. Age-related changes in vitreous mobility as measured by video B scan ultrasound. *Exp Eye Res* 2002;74(2):173–80.
5. Foos, R. Y. and Wheeler, N. C. Vitreoretinal juncture: Synchysis senilis and posterior vitreous detachment. *Ophthalmology* 1982;89(12):1502–12.

6. Hikichi, T., Takahashi, M., Trempe, C. L. and Schepens, C. L. Relationship between premacular cortical vitreous defects and idiopathic premacular fibrosis. *Retina* 1995;15(5):413–6.

7. Hikichi, T., Trempe, C. L. and Schepens, C. L. Posterior vitreous detachment as a risk factor for retinal detachment. *Ophthalmology* 1995;102(4):527–8.

8. Sebag, J. Abnormalities of human vitreous structure in diabetes. *Graefes Arch Clin Exp Ophthalmol* 1993;231(5):257–60.

9. Morita, H., Funata, M. and Tokoro, T. A clinical study of the development of posterior vitreous detachment in high myopia. *Retina* 1995;15(2):117–24.

10. Yonemoto, J., Ideta, H., Sasaki, K. et al. The age of onset of posterior vitreous detachment. *Graefes Arch Clin Exp Ophthalmol* 1994;232(2):67–70.

11. Akiba, J. Prevalence of posterior vitreous detachment in high myopia. *Ophthalmology* 1993;100(9):1384–8.

12. Chuo, J. Y., Lee, T. Y., Hollands, H. et al. Risk factors for posterior vitreous detachment: A case-control study. *Am J Ophthalmol* 2006;142(6):931–7.

13. Mahroo, O. A., Mitry, D., Williamson, T. H. et al. Exploring sex and laterality imbalances in patients undergoing laser retinopexy. *JAMA Ophthalmol* 2015;133(11):1334–6.

14. Hikichi, T., Hirokawa, H., Kado, M. et al. Comparison of the prevalence of posterior vitreous detachment in whites and Japanese. *Ophthalmic Surg* 1995;26(1):39–43.

15. Weiss, H. and Tasman, W. S. Rhegmatogenous retinal detachments in blacks. *Ann Ophthalmol* 1978;10(6):799–806.

16. Foos, R. Y., Simons, K. B. and Wheeler, N. C. Comparison of lesions predisposing to rhegmatogenous retinal detachment by race of subjects. *Am J Ophthalmol* 1983;96(5):644–9.

17. Hikichi, T. and Yoshida, A. Time course of development of posterior vitreous detachment in the fellow eye after development in the first eye. *Ophthalmology* 2004;111(9):1705–7.

18. Novak, M. A. and Welch, R. B. Complications of acute symptomatic posterior vitreous detachment. *Am J Ophthalmol* 1984;97(3):308–14.

19. Kado, M., Jalkh, A. E., Yoshida, A. et al. Vitreous changes and macular edema in central retinal vein occlusion. *Ophthalmic Surg* 1990;21(8):544–9.

20. Unal, M. and Peyman, G. A. The efficacy of plasminogen-urokinase combination in inducing posterior vitreous detachment. *Retina* 2000;20(1):69–75.

21. Hesse, L., Nebeling, B., Schroeder, B. et al. Induction of posterior vitreous detachment in rabbits by intravitreal injection of tissue plasminogen activator following cryopexy. *Exp Eye Res* 2000;70(1):31–9.

22. Kakehashi, A., Ueno, N. and Chakrabarti, B. Molecular mechanisms of photochemically induced posterior vitreous detachment. *Ophthalmic Res* 1994;26(1):51–9.

23. Hikichi, T., Yanagiya, N., Kado, M. et al. Posterior vitreous detachment induced by injection of plasmin and sulfur hexafluoride in the rabbit vitreous. *Retina* 1999;19(1):55–8.

24. Verstraeten, T. C., Chapman, C., Hartzer, M. et al. Pharmacologic induction of posterior vitreous detachment in the rabbit. *Arch Ophthalmol* 1993;111(6):849–54.

25. Harooni, M., McMillan, T. and Refojo, M. Efficacy and safety of enzymatic posterior vitreous detachment by intravitreal injection of hyaluronidase. *Retina* 1998;18(1):16–22.

26. Tezel, T. H., Del Priore, L. V. and Kaplan, H. J. Posterior vitreous detachment with dispase. *Retina* 1998;18(1):7–15.

27. Kang, S. W., Hyung, S. M., Choi, M. Y. and Lee J. Induction of vitreolysis and vitreous detachment with hyaluronidase and perfluoropropane gas. *Korean J Ophthalmol* 1995;9(2):69–78.

28. Stalmans, P., Benz, M. S., Gandorfer, A. et al. Enzymatic vitreolysis with ocriplasmin for vitreomacular traction and macular holes. *N Engl J Med* 2012;367(7):606–15.

29. Akiba, J., Ishiko, S. and Yoshida, A. Variations of Weiss's ring. *Retina* 2001;21(3):243–6.

30. Kakehashi, A., Inoda, S., Shimizu, Y. et al. Predictive value of floaters in the diagnosis of posterior vitreous detachment. *Am J Ophthalmol* 1998;125(1):113–5.

31. Uchino, E., Uemuram, A. and Ohba, N. Initial stages of posterior vitreous detachment in healthy eyes of older persons evaluated by optical coherence tomography. *Arch Ophthalmol* 2001;119(10):1475–9.

32. Purkinje, J. E. *Beiträge zur Kenntniss des Sehens in subjectiver Hinsicht* (*Contributions to the Knowledge of Vision in Its Subjective Aspect*). Prague: J. G. Calve, 1819.

33. Moore, R. F. Subjective 'lightning streaks'. *Br J Ophthalmol* 1935;19:545–7.

34. Moore, R. F. Subjective 'lightning flashes'. *Am J Ophthalmol* 1940;23:1255–60.

35. Moore, R. F. Subjective 'lightning streaks'. *Br J Ophthalmol* 1947;31:46–50.

36. Verhoeff, F. H. Moore's subjective 'lightning streaks'. *Trans Am Acad Ophthalmol Soc* 1941;39:220–6.

37. Berens, C., Cholst, M., Emmerich, R. and McGrath, H. Moore's lightning streaks: A discussion of their innocuousness. *Trans Am Acad Ophthalmol Soc* 1954;52:35–58.

38. Williamson, T. H., Watt, L. and Mokete, B. Black or negative flashes in posterior vitreous detachment a transient symptom before lightning flashes commence. *Eye* 2009;23(6):1477.

39. Goodfellow, J. F., Mokete, B. and Williamson, T. H. Discriminate characteristics of photopsia in posterior vitreous detachment, retinal tears and retinal detachment. *Ophthalmic Physiol Opt* 2010;30(1):20–3.

40. van Overdam, K. A., Bettink-Remeijer, M. W., Mulder, P. G. and van Meurs, J. C. Symptoms predictive for the later development of retinal breaks. *Arch Ophthalmol* 2001;119(10):1483–6.

41. Sharma, S., Walker, R., Brown, G. C. and Cruess, A. F. The importance of qualitative vitreous examination in patients with acute posterior vitreous detachment. *Arch Ophthalmol* 1999;117(3):343–6.

42. Hikichi, T. and Trempe, C. L. Relationship between floaters, light flashes, or both, and complications of posterior vitreous detachment. *Am J Ophthalmol* 1994;117(5):593–8.

43. Serpetopoulos, C. Optical explanation of the gradual disappearance of flying dots in posterior vitreous detachment. *Surv Ophthalmol* 1997;42(1):92–4.

44. Hollands, H., Johnson, D., Brox, A. C. et al. Acute-onset floaters and flashes: Is this patient at risk for retinal detachment? *JAMA* 2009;302(20):2243–9.

45. Tanner, V., Harle, D., Tan, J. et al. Acute posterior vitreous detachment: The predictive value of vitreous pigment and symptomatology. *Br J Ophthalmol* 2000;84(11):1264–8.

46. Dayan, M. R., Jayamanne, D. G., Andrews, R. M. and Griffiths, P. G. Flashes and floaters as predictors of vitreoretinal pathology: Is follow-up necessary for posterior vitreous detachment? *Eye* 1996;10 (Pt 4):456–8.

47. Byer, N. E. Natural history of posterior vitreous detachment with early management as the premier line of defense against retinal detachment. *Ophthalmology* 1994;101(9):1503–13.

48. Brod, R. D., Lightman, D. A., Packer, A. J. and Saras, H. P. Correlation between vitreous pigment granules and retinal breaks in eyes with acute posterior vitreous detachment. *Ophthalmology* 1991;98(9):1366–9.

49. Coffee, R. E., Westfall, A. C., Davis, G. H. et al. Symptomatic posterior vitreous detachment and the incidence of delayed retinal breaks: Case series and meta-analysis. *Am J Ophthalmol* 2007;144(3):409–13.

50. Katz, B. and Hoyt, W. F. Intrapapillary and peripapillary hemorrhage in young patients with incomplete posterior vitreous detachment: Signs of vitreopapillary traction. *Ophthalmology* 1995;102(2):349–54.

51. Roberts, T. V. and Gregory-Roberts, J. C. Optic disc haemorrhages in posterior vitreous detachment. *Aust NZ J Ophthalmol* 1991;19(1):61–3.

52. Cibis, G. W., Watzke, R. C. and Chua, J. Retinal hemorrhages in posterior vitreous detachment. *Am J Ophthalmol* 1975;80(6):1043–6.

53. Schachat, A. P. and Sommer, A. Macular hemorrhages associated with posterior vitreous detachment. *Am J Ophthalmol* 1986;102(5):647–9.

54. Richardson, P. S., Benson, M. T. and Kirkby, G. R. The posterior vitreous detachment clinic: Do new retinal breaks develop in the six weeks following an isolated symptomatic posterior vitreous detachment? *Eye* 1999;13 (Pt 2):237–40.

55. Williams, K. M., Watt, L. and Williamson, T. H. Acute symptomatic posterior vitreous detachment and delayed retinal breaks. *Acta Ophthalmol* 2011;89(1):e100–1.

56. Byer, N. E. What happens to untreated asymptomatic retinal breaks, and are they affected by posterior vitreous detachment? *Ophthalmology* 1998;105(6):1045–9.

57. Byer, N. E. Subclinical retinal detachment resulting from asymptomatic retinal breaks: Prognosis for progression and regression. *Ophthalmology* 2001;108(8):1499–503.

58. Byer, N. E. The natural history of asymptomatic retinal breaks. *Ophthalmology* 1982;89(9):1033–9.

59. Murakami-Nagasako, F. and Ohba, N. Phakic retinal detachment associated with atrophic hole of lattice degeneration of the retina. *Graefes Arch Clin Exp Ophthalmol* 1983;220(4):175–8.

60. Semes, L. P., Holland, W. C. and Likens, E. G. Prevalence and laterality of lattice retinal degeneration within a primary eye care population. *Optometry* 2001;72(4):247–50.

61. Celorio, J. M. and Pruett, R. C. Prevalence of lattice degeneration and its relation to axial length in severe myopia. *Am J Ophthalmol* 1991;111(1):20–3.

62. Byer, N. E. Long-term natural history of lattice degeneration of the retina. *Ophthalmology* 1989;96(9):1396–401.

63. Benson, W. E., Morse, P. H. and Nantawan, P. Late complications following cryotherapy of lattice degeneration. *Am J Ophthalmol* 1977;84(4):514–6.

64. Shukla, M. and Ahuja, O. P. A possible relationship between lattice and snail track degenerations of the retina. *Am J Ophthalmol* 1981;92(4):482–5.

65. Lewis, H., Straatsma, B. R. and Foos, R. Y, Lightfoot DO: Reticular degeneration of the pigment epithelium. *Ophthalmology* 1985;92(11):1485–95.

66. Humphrey, W. T., Carlson, R. E. and Valone, J. A. Jr. Senile reticular pigmentary degeneration. *Am J Ophthalmol* 1984;98(6):717–22.

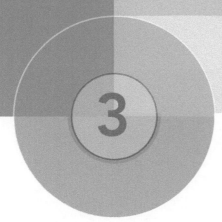

Vitreous haemorrhage

3

Vitreous haemorrhage (VH) complicates disorders of the retina and will often cause severe reduction of vision. A small quantity of haemorrhage is required to reduce the vision. Occasionally, a good visual acuity can be recorded because the patient can momentarily visualise the test chart through a clear section of vitreous before the opacified vitreous obscures the vision again. The haemorrhage may be situated as follows:

- In the gel of the vitreous (intragel)
- Behind a detached gel (retrohyaloid)

There may be associated haemorrhage under the internal limiting membrane (ILM) and under the retina or in the choroid (Figures 3.1 and 3.2).

AETIOLOGY

- A primary cause of spontaneous VH is retinal neovascularisation secondary to retinal ischaemia (most commonly, diabetic retinopathy or retinal vein occlusion). This usually is associated with PVD; i.e. the mobile vitreous tears the fragile new blood vessels, in which case, a subhyaloid haemorrhage is common. The vitreous may be attached if the blood vessels burst either spontaneously or during a period of raised systemic blood pressure (e.g. during isometric exertion).
- VH from retinal tears associated with PVD requires most urgent management.
- Haemorrhage elsewhere in the eye will often disperse into the vitreous cavity, e.g. suprachoroidal blood in trauma, subretinal blood secondary to choroidal neovascularisation (CNV) or blood under the ILM in Terson's syndrome.
- Other common causes of vitreous cavity haemorrhage are retinal macroaneurysm (often the vitreous is attached).
- VH from PVD without retinal tear formation should be diagnosed with care and only assumed once other causes have been excluded.
- In infants, haemorrhage from retinopathy of prematurity is possible.

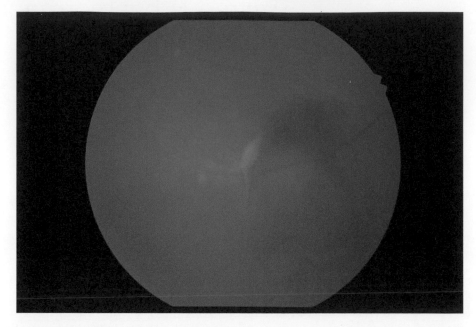

Figure 3.1 Resolution of subretinal haemorrhage may leave subretinal scar tissue.

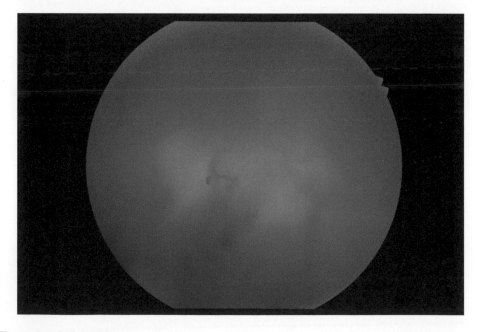

Figure 3.2 Diffused VH.

- In children overall, 73% of cases are due to manifest or occult trauma; other common causes are regressed retinopathy of prematurity.[1] Shaken baby syndrome from non-accidental injury should be considered in bilateral VH. Rare causes are juvenile retinoschisis, familial exudative vitreoretinopathy, intermediate uveitis, other uveitis and tumours.
- Sub-ILM bleeds are rare and seen in Terson's syndrome, Valsalva-related haemorrhage (forced breath holding), blood dyscrasia and trauma.[2] Terson's syndrome has been reported in 8–14% of patients with subarachnoid haemorrhage.[3]

CAUSES[4–10]

- Diabetic retinopathy
- Branch retinal vein occlusion (BRVO)
- Retinal tear and RRD
- Choroidal neovascular membrane
- Macroaneurysm
- PVD
- Trauma
- Sickle cell retinopathy
- Central retinal vein occlusion (CRVO)
- Terson's syndrome
- Retinal vasculitis
- Intermediate uveitis
- Retinoschisis
- Needle-stick injury
- Tumour (vasoproliferative)
- Familial exudative vitreoretinopathy
- Retinal telangiectasia
- Valsalva manoeuvre

NATURAL HISTORY

The blood in the vitreous gel initially forms a localised clot, but subsequent fibrinolysis (break-down of the clot) causes the dispersion of the haemorrhage throughout the gel. During haemolysis, biconcave erythrocytes lose most of their enclosed haemoglobin and change to spheroidal erythroclasts. The degradation of the released haemoglobin produces pigments, which often stain the gel with an ochre-yellow or orange colour. In very severe old haemorrhage, an 'ochre membrane' is seen.

The mechanisms of spontaneous absorption of VH are as follows:

- Phagocytosis by macrophages
- Outflow of cells through the trabecular meshwork
- Syneretic disintegration of the gel

Cells in the trabecular meshwork can reduce aqueous drainage causing raised intra-ocular pressure (IOP) and 'erythroclastic glaucoma'. Another rare consequence of vitreous

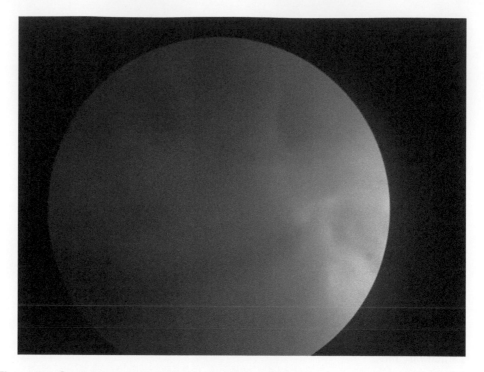

Figure 3.3 Severe VH in a patient who is on warfarin systemically.

haemorrhage later on after absorption of most of the blood is 'synchisis scintillans', a localised form of cholesterolosis bulbi. It is characterised by the presence of cholesterol crystals in the vitreous cavity, which tend to sediment inferiorly (Figure 3.3).

ERYTHROCLASTIC GLAUCOMA

The macrophages, which remove the haemorrhage, clog up the trabecular meshwork causing a rise in IOP. If a vitreous haemorrhage is left in the eye for weeks or months, glaucoma is an occasional risk. If undetected and untreated, glaucomatous damage to the optic disc can result. Therefore, the eye with vitreous haemorrhage will require periodic IOP checks.

INVESTIGATION

The priority with vitreous haemorrhage is determining the aetiology because some causes require immediate intervention. The cause in many cases can be determined from the history of the patient:

- Diabetic retinopathy
- BRVO with previous symptoms
  - Previous loss of vision 1 year ago/laser
- Trauma
  - Traumatic history
- CRVO
  - Loss of vision 2 years ago

- Terson's syndrome
  - Headache, neurological signs and symptoms
- Needle-stick injury
  - Careless anaesthesia/intravitreal injection
- Sickle cell
  - Race, past medical history and blood tests
- Retinal vasculitis
  - Previous systemic treatment (Figure 3.4)

Some patients will have no prior history:

- BRVO previously asymptomatic
- Choroidal neovascular membrane
  - Often the presenting complaint in these patients with or without signs of age-related macular degeneration (AMD) in the other eye
- Macroaneurysm
- PVD with or without retinal tears
  - Flashes and floaters may have been present but are inconclusive clinical features
- Retinal vasculitis
- Intermediate uveitis
  - Beware of the 20-year-old patient with vitreous haemorrhage; they may have had undiagnosed panuveitis. Ask for a history of floaters prior to the onset of the vitreous haemorrhage.
- Retinoschisis
- Tumour

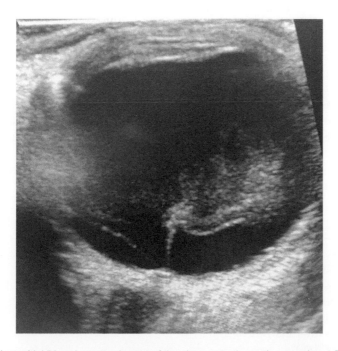

Figure 3.4 Patient with VH and an attachment of the vitreous to the optic nerve head. The most common cause of this is neovascularisation of the optic disc; in fact, this patient had tuberculosis and retinal vasculitis.

If the vitreous haemorrhage is mild, it may be possible to see the cause with slit lamp biomicroscopy and a 90D lens or with an indirect ophthalmoscope. Scleral indentation may be required to exclude retinal tears. If a view is not available, ultrasound is the mainstay of investigation.

ULTRASOUND

Referral for ultrasound will help determine the diagnosis but will usually require specialised input to interpret.

- A sinuous continuous high echo, which starts at the ora serrata and ends around the optic nerve head, is typical of detached retina. In contrast, a PVD will move with a more rapid and flimsy action.
- The flap of a retinal tear is observed attached to the peripheral vitreous. A sensitivity of 56% has been estimated for detecting retinal tears on ultrasound in eyes with VH.[11]
- Attachment of the vitreous to the disc is present with new disc vessels in diabetes or BRVO.
- Diffuse increased echo behind the gel indicates retrohyaloid blood. Retinal detachments have clear fluid on ultrasound behind their echogenic signal, i.e. subretinal fluid in the subretinal space.
- If the vitreous is still attached, this may aid in diagnosis, suggesting diabetic retinopathy or an unusual cause such as Terson's syndrome (Chapter 11).
- The focal attachments of an otherwise detached vitreous can be helpful, e.g. the vitreous attached to new vessels at the disc or elsewhere, tractional retinal detachments or incarceration sites in trauma or needle-stick injury.
- Other conditions will provide clues of their own. Choroidal neovascular membranes that bleed tend to produce severe subretinal haemorrhage, which can be seen as a dense immobile craggy mass at the posterior pole. The patient will usually have signs of high-risk AMD in the other eye, e.g. soft drusen or disciform scar.
- Tumours have their own characteristic shapes, e.g. collar stud melanoma. Colour Doppler imaging helps by demonstrating a tumour circulation in elevated, e.g. metastases and malignant melanomas. Vasoproliferative tumours are flatter and more difficult to detect with Doppler.
- Retinoschisis provides a thin dome-shaped peripheral elevation. X-linked retinoschisis is particularly associated with VH in the young.

ULTRASOUND FEATURES

- Vitreous detached or not
  - If attached, it is not a retinal tear!
  - Subhyaloid haemorrhage is common when the vitreous is detached and delineates the posterior of the vitreous. Haemorrhage in this position is usually liquefied and mobile (Figure 3.5).
- Evidence of neovascularisation
  - BRVO or CRVO.
  - But beware of the posterior retinal break which can be attached to the gel and look like posterior neovascularisation.

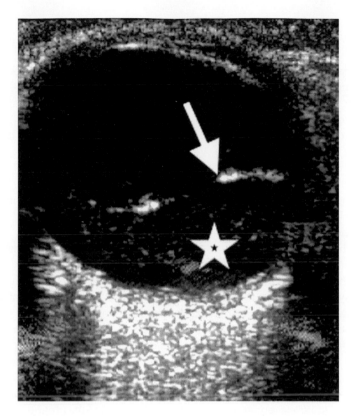

Figure 3.5 Ultrasound of an eye with subhyaloid haemorrhage (*star*). The posterior vitreous face is seen at the arrow.

- Subretinal haemorrhage
  - Large craggy mass under the retina.
  - CNV can be posterior or peripheral.
  - Haemorrhage in this position is clotted and solidified.
- Management
  - Do you have a retinal tear?
    - Can you wait?
    - Does the eye need an operation?
  - You cannot afford to miss the threat of a retinal detachment.
    - Risk of retinal tear going on to RRD
    - Risk of proliferative vitreoretinopathy in RRD with VH

REFERRAL

This depends on the whether the cause is known or not. Unfortunately, this information is not always discernable. In a diabetic patient with diabetic retinopathy, the vast majority of cases are due to the retinopathy. Referral will vary depending on the retinopathy status (see Chapter 7).

VITREOUS HAEMORRHAGE NON-DIABETIC

- History
  - If you can determine from the history the cause of the haemorrhage, you can refer accordingly, e.g. a history of retinal vein occlusion, trauma and sickle cell retinopathy.
- No history
  - Pathology seen
    - You may be able to see the cause and therefore act accordingly, but more often, the retina is obscured.
  - No pathology seen
    - Ultrasound is required, and for this, referral is required most often. The referral needs to be emergency (24 hours) because a retinal tear or detachment has not yet been excluded.
  - On ultrasound
    - If the vitreous is attached, it is very unlikely to be a retinal tear from PVD, and therefore, urgent vitrectomy is less likely to be required.
    - If the vitreous is detached, there is a risk of retinal tear; however, the ultrasound may identify a mass in the eye or new vessels seen as an attachment of the vitreous to the optic disc (for disc neovascularisation) or elsewhere at the posterior pole (neovascularisation elsewhere; care needs to be taken not to confuse this with a posterior retinal tear).
    - If a retinal tear or a retinal detachment or nothing else is identified other than the PVD, the patient needs to be taken for an urgent vitrectomy to clear out the blood and inspect the retina. In this circumstance, a significant group will be found to have a retinal tear which would have risked the progression to retinal detachment.

MEDICOLEGAL CASE

A patient attends her optician with reduced vision in one eye. The optician notes the description of reduction in vision and large pupil. The vision in each eye is recorded as normal. The eye is examined, and a normal optic nerve and normal visual fields are recorded. The optician refers to an FP.

The patient is seen by the FP on the same day. The FP refers the patient to the local hospital as a routine referral but noting the fixed pupil. There is delay in the set-up of the patient's appointment at the hospital. The FP realizes there is delay some months later and sends a further letter, but the patient is not seen until months after the initial referral.

On attendance at the hospital, the patient has no perception of light in the eye and is found to have vitreous haemorrhage and neovascular glaucoma. The pressure in the eye is highly elevated. The optic nerve has a full glaucomatous cup.

The patient is found to have an ischaemic central retinal vein occlusion resulting in vitreous haemorrhage and neovascular glaucoma.

Errors were made by the FP, who did not recognize the serious clinical sign of dilated pupil. The initial finding of good vision in the eye may have falsely reassured the FP that a routine referral was safe. This led to failure to refer promptly for review.

After considerable delay, the patient was seen, but irreversible glaucomatous damage had already occurred.

The patient was diagnosed with left neovascular glaucoma, with VH. The patient had cyclo-diode laser to try to treat the glaucoma.

It is likely that the patient had an ischaemic CRVO resulting in VH and neovascular glaucoma. Errors were made by the family practitioners not recognizing the serious clinical signs of dilated and unresponsive pupil and reduced vision and failing to refer promptly for review. After considerable delay, the patient was seen, but irreversible glaucomatous damage had already occurred.

REFERENCES

1. Spirn, M. J., Lynn, M. J. and Hubbard, G. B. III. Vitreous hemorrhage in children. *Ophthalmology* 2006;113(5):848–52.
2. De Maeyer, K., Van Ginderdeuren, R., Postelmans, L. et al. Sub-inner limiting membrane haemorrhage: Causes and treatment with vitrectomy. *Br J Ophthalmol* 2007;91(7):869–72.
3. Garweg, J. G. and Koerner, F. Outcome indicators for vitrectomy in Terson syndrome. *Acta Ophthalmol* 2009;87(2):222–6.
4. Lauer, A. K., Smith, J. R., Robertson, J. E. and Rosenbaum, J. T. Vitreous hemorrhage is a common complication of pediatric pars planitis. *Ophthalmology* 2002;109(1):95–8.
5. Zhao, P., Hayashi, H., Oshima, K. et al. Vitrectomy for macular hemorrhage associated with retinal arterial macroaneurysm. *Ophthalmology* 2000;107(3):613–7.
6. Kuhn, F., Morris, R., Witherspoon, C. D. and Mester, V. Terson syndrome: Results of vitrectomy and the significance of vitreous hemorrhage in patients with subarachnoid hemorrhage. *Ophthalmology* 1998;105(3):472–7.
7. Dana, M. R., Werner, M. S., Viana, M. A. and Shapiro, M. J. Spontaneous and traumatic vitreous hemorrhage. *Ophthalmology* 1993;100(9):1377–83.
8. el Baba, F., Jarrett, W. H., Harbin, T. S. Jr. et al. Massive hemorrhage complicating age-related macular degeneration: Clinicopathologic correlation and role of anticoagulants. *Ophthalmology* 1986;93(12):1581–92.
9. Lean, J. S. and Gregor, Z. The acute vitreous haemorrhage. *Br J Ophthalmol* 1980;64(7):469–71.
10. Sarrafizadeh, R., Hassan, T. S., Ruby, A. J. et al. Incidence of retinal detachment and visual outcome in eyes presenting with posterior vitreous separation and dense fundus-obscuring vitreous hemorrhage. *Ophthalmology* 2001;108(12):2273–8.
11. Tan, H. S., Mura, M. and Bijl, H. M. Early vitrectomy for vitreous hemorrhage associated with retinal tears. *Am J Ophthalmol* 2010;150(4):529–33.

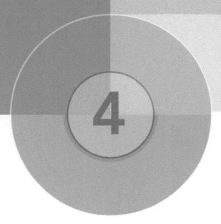

Rhegmatogenous retinal detachment

4

Strictly speaking, *retinal detachment* is a misnomer. The term denotes separation of the neuroepithelium from the pigment epithelium (rather than the detachment of the retina, which consists of the neuroepithelium and the RPE, from the choroid). The incidence is approximately 1:10,000,[1] and presentation is more common in affluent populations and, possibly, males.[2] In middle-aged patients, the incidence is approximately 1:300. Blacks are probably less affected than whites are[3] (Figure 4.1).

The most common cause of retinal detachment is the formation of a 'break' or full-thickness discontinuity in the neuroepithelium, which allows the fluid from the vitreous cavity into the subretinal space via the break, creating RRD. Classically, breaks are subdivided into *tears* (secondary to dynamic vitreoretinal traction) and *holes* (secondary to localised retinal disintegration or atrophy) (Figure 4.2).

TEARS WITH POSTERIOR VITREOUS DETACHMENT

Most retinal tears occur in association with spontaneous PVD by the operation of *dynamic vitreous traction*. This term denotes the transmission of rotational energy (generated by the saccadic contraction of the extra ocular muscles) to the vitreous gel through the coats of the eye (sclera, choroid and retina). While the vitreous remains attached to the retina, this energy transmission is dispersed throughout the total area of vitreoretinal contact. After PVD, however, the forces produce considerable movement in the posterior gel. The vitreous base provides the centre of energy while the posterior vitreous responds to the energy by accelerating into a violent movement (Figures 4.3 and 4.4).

If there is any area of 'abnormal' adhesion of the retina to the gel, the movement of the gel exerts considerable dynamic traction on the retina, which may rip as a result, producing a U-shaped tear of the retina. The base of the tongue of the torn retina, which produces the *U*, is anteriorly placed because the vitreous separates first posteriorly, tearing the retina at a point of adhesion, and the action of the vitreous extends the tear anteriorly towards the vitreous base. If the flap of the tear separates completely from the retina, the piece of avulsed neurosensory retina is seen attached to the posterior vitreous membrane as an operculum and a round tear are produced (Figure 4.5).

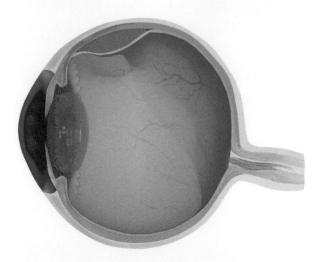

Figure 4.1 Fluid from the vitreous cavity can enter into the subretinal space through the retinal break, creating RRD.

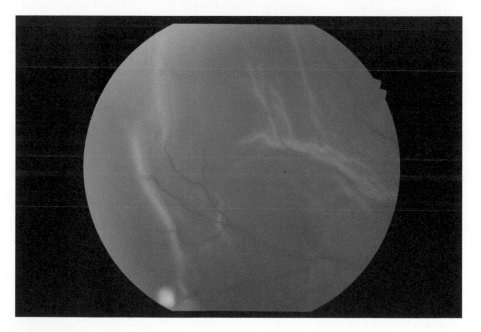

Figure 4.2 Detached retina.

Haemorrhage from the rupture of a blood vessel that crosses a U tear may produce a 'tadpole' floater or a shower of floaters. Floaters may also be seen from the PVD and photopsia (flashing lights) from traction on the retina.

The vitreous is adherent to the rim of lattice lesions. U tears in lattice therefore tear along the posterior border of the lattice and then extend anteriorly around the edge of the lesion.

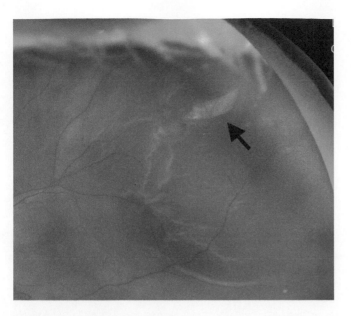

Figure 4.3 Large retinal tear in retinal detachment.

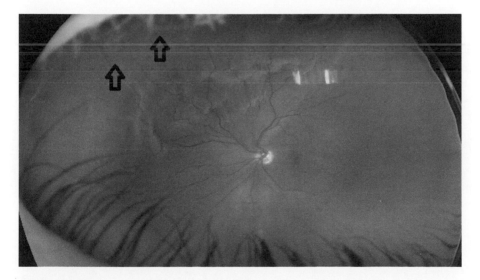

Figure 4.4 Two retinal tears can be seen in the periphery of this retinal detachment.

Multiple tiny flap breaks at the posterior border of the vitreous base are particularly associated with aphakia (no lens) or pseudophakia (artificial lens). The reasons for this are not clear, but cataract extraction alters the architecture of vitreous through the loss of the posterior bulge of the crystalline lens into the anterior vitreous, and this may alter the separation of the vitreous in the eye (Figures 4.6 and 4.7).

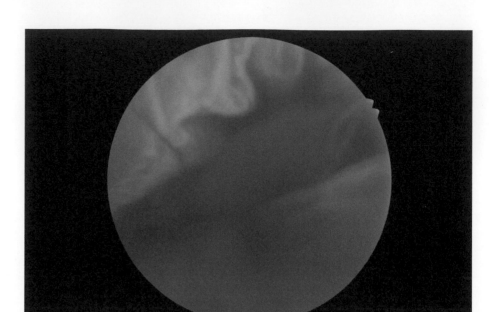

Figure 4.5 Bullous retinal detachment.

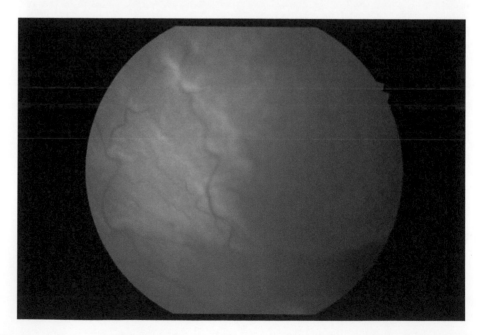

Figure 4.6 Bullous retinal detachments where the retina is highly elevated, usually arising from retinal breaks in the superior portion of the eye. These will spread faster than shallow retinal detachments, spreading upwards from the inferior retina.

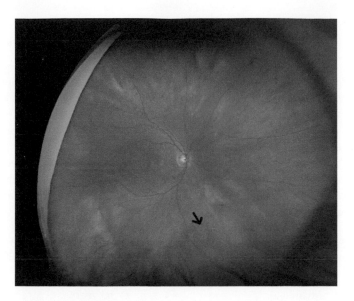

Figure 4.7 Inferior retinal detachment.

BREAKS WITHOUT POSTERIOR VITREOUS DETACHMENT

RRD may be produced without PVD by atrophic retinal holes often in young myopic patients (these patients are more likely to be female, 64%, with bilateral pathology in 83%[4]) or by retinal dialysis at the ora serrata. Both conditions usually produce a slow onset of retinal detachment, which may only be noticed during coincidental examination of the eye or symptomatically by the patient when the fovea detaches. Atrophic holes are often equatorial, associated with lattice degeneration and myopia, and found in 20–40-year-old patients.[5] The vast majority will not cause retinal detachment, and prophylactic therapy is generally regarded as unnecessary. The recruitment of fluid in a round hole detachment probably occurs by the connection of the hole to the fluid-filled lacunae in the vitreous. This may cause a stepped increase in the detachment with multiple pigmentary demarcation lines in a chronic-looking retinal detachment.

Retinal dialyses are ellipsoid separations of the retina at the ora serrata that are usually situated inferotemporally. They differ from U tears because the gel is attached to the posterior rather than the anterior margin of the break and the PVD is absent. The fluid in these retinal detachments may come from the anterior chamber.

NATURAL HISTORY

- Most retinal detachments if untreated will progress to totality or near totality rapidly over days. The visual loss is profound and commences with peripheral visual field loss (like a curtain or shadow) followed by loss of the central vision. Potential recovery of vision after successful surgery reduces as the weeks go by.
- The retina is thickened and less transparent when it is detached.
- If the retina remains detached for many months, it becomes progressively atrophic.
- The longer the retina remains detached, the higher the risk of a scarring response and proliferative vitreoretinopathy (PVR) (see the 'Risk of PUR' section).

CHRONIC RRD

In a longstanding subtotal retinal detachment, a 'high-water mark' or pigment demarcation line of retinal pigment hyperplasia may appear in the flat retina adjacent to the detached retina. Multiple high-water marks in detached retina indicate the recurrent extension of the detachment and are more often seen in slower onset detachments associated with round holes or dialyses. Other indices of longstanding detachment include retinal cysts (secondary retinoschisis),[6] oxalate crystals on the macula[7] and peripheral neovascularisation.

Very rarely, the retina reattaches spontaneously, sometimes leaving pigmented chorioretinal changes, but most often, surgery is required to reattach the retina. After successful surgery, the rods recover their function surprisingly well, and any visual field defect disappears. If the fovea has been involved, recovery of function of the cones is good if the detachment is treated quickly (within 1 week of onset). After prolonged detachment of the fovea, the central vision may be permanently impaired despite successful reattachment (Figure 4.8).

- Descriptive statistics for a north European population[8]

• Mean age	• 53 years
• Bilateral	• 10%
• Lattice degeneration	• 15%
• More dialyses	• <20 years old
• Tears = atrophic holes	• 20–40 years old
• Predominantly tears	• >40 years old
• Bilateral simultaneous[9]	• 2.3%

The characteristics of the eye in a group of patients with RRD are shown in Table 4.1.[2] The chance of RRD in the fellow eye is 12%, with 12% chance of retinopexy to a tear.[10]

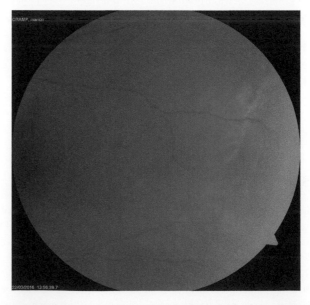

Figure 4.8 Edge of a chronic retinal detachment showing pigmentation along the junction of the attached and detached retina.

Table 4.1 RRD characteristics

Variable	Ratio (%)
Sex	
Female	39.9
Male	60.1
Eye	
Left	44.4
Right	55.6
Lens status	
Normal crystalline lens	38.8
Cortical cataract	5.8
Mixed cataract	2.6
Nuclear sclerotic cataract	21.1
Posterior chamber Intraocular lens	29.9
Posterior subcapsular cataract	1.8
Success of surgery	
Primary	87.0
Secondary	10.2
Fail	2.8
Operation	
Drainage, air, cryotherapy and explant	0.4
Non-drain (cryotherapy and buckle)	9.6
PPV	90.1
Fovea off	56.3
Breaks	
Nil	0.4
Mixed	19.3
Round	10.4
U tears	69.9
PVD	89.5
VH	
Mild	7.8
Moderate	3.4
Severe	0.7
Quadrants of RRD	
1	24.4
2	35.5
3	26.9
4	13.2
B PVR	8.4
PVR (PVR, b and c)	14.2

CLINICAL FEATURES

The patient may experience the following symptoms:

- Flashes and floaters (indicating PVD with or without VH): Some slow onset retinal detachments will produce the symptom of a slow flashing light (often moving like a tail of a slow comet) lasting a few seconds and situated in the visual field appropriate to the leading edge of subretinal fluid (SRF).

- Visual field loss in the form of a curtain coming over the peripheral vision: The visual field loss is opposite the site of detachment, e.g. an inferonasal loss indicates a supero-temporal retinal detachment. The deficit spreads from the periphery to the central vision at a variable rate from a few hours, to days, to weeks.
- When the fovea detaches, there is loss of central vision, with the fovea just off the visual acuity may vary from 20/40 to 20/200.
- As the fovea lifts, the patient may experience distortion of vision.
- When the macula is fully detached, the vision may be 20/200 to hand movements.

ANTERIOR SEGMENT SIGNS

- A few cells and some flare can be seen in the anterior chamber. Rarely, a severe anterior uveitis occurs perhaps indicating a high risk of PVR.
- IOP is often lower than the fellow eye. Occasionally, a high IOP can be produced by the blockage of the trabecular meshwork by the remnants of receptor outer segments (Schwartz's syndrome).[11,12]
- Iris neovascularisation has occasionally been described, which reverses after the resolution of the RRD.[13]

SIGNS IN THE VITREOUS

Retinal tear formation is usually associated with the release of retinal pigment epithelial cells into the vitreous cavity. The presence of pigment cells in the retrolental gel (Shafer's sign)[14] in a phakic eye strongly implies the presence of a retinal break. The differentiation of these cells into fibroblast-like cells and synthesis of new collagen within the gel and on the posterior hyaloid interface results in the stiffness of the gel. An early sign of this process is seen when the cells change from diffused single cells to groups or 'clumps' of cells in the gel. Such changes are frequently associated with fibrosis on the retinal surface in PVR. VH caused by the rupture of a retinal blood vessel may obscure the view of the retina and breaks. Suspect that any patient with VH of unknown aetiology has a retinal tear or detachment.

SUBRETINAL FLUID ACCUMULATION

The separation of the neuroepithelium from the pigment epithelium occurs first around the break. Progressively, more SRF is recruited from the vitreous cavity (from the retrohyaloid space or from syneretic gel), increasing the area and elevation of retinal separation. Progression has been estimated at 1.8 disc diameters per day.[15] If the globe is completely immobilised at an early stage, the retina may partially or even completely reattach suggesting that three mechanisms may be implicated.

- Movement of the eye (and the resultant vitreous gel movement) causes the extension of the retinal detachment through the action of dynamic vitreoretinal traction.
- The movement of the gel induces fluid currents in the vitreous cavity, which forcefully elevate the neurosensory retina.[16]

- Gravity encourages the spread of the relatively dense SRF. This causes a pattern of spread of SRF first described by Lincoff and Gieser[17] that may be used by the clinician to aid the localisation of a retinal break.
  - A tear between 11 o'clock and 1 o'clock causes a retinal detachment, which becomes total soon after its onset.
  - Tears above the horizontal meridian (3 to 9 o'clock) produce subtotal detachments. Fluid is recruited progressing downwards on the same side as the tear at first and then upwards on the opposite side of the disc (but to a level lower than that on the side of the tear).
  - Inferior SRF from a superior tear tends to separate partially into two bullae with a cleft or 'cleavage' of less-elevated retina in the six o'clock meridian.
  - A break located below the horizontal meridian tends to accumulate fluid more slowly compared with that descending from above. The upper limits of the detachment form convex curved edges on each side, the higher edge indicating the side of the break. Bullae are not seen with inferior breaks.
  - Occasionally, a small anterior and superior tear leaks fluid down the post-oral retina causing an inferior retinal detachment. Therefore, inferior retinal detachment can occur from both superior and inferior tears.

SRF accumulates more quickly if the fluid is recruited from the retrohyaloid space (e.g. via a U tear after PVD) compared with breaks occurring without PVD (e.g. atrophic holes and dialyses). In the latter, the potential recruitment of fluid from syneretic gel may be limited by the size of the lacuna in the gel (Figure 4.9).

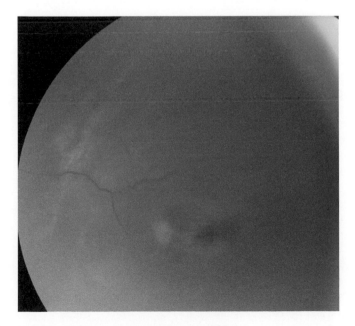

Figure 4.9 Operculated hole in an area of retinal detachment.

RETINAL BREAK PATTERNS IN RRD

Breaks are more common temporally and superiorly than nasally or inferiorly in PVD-related RRD (Table 4.2). See the next chapter for more details.

MACULA OFF OR ON

When the fovea of the macula detaches (usually called *macula off*), the chances of return of full central vision is reduced particularly after the first week of detachment. For this reason, surgeons prefer to operate when the fovea is attached. It is important to refer a patient with a macula-on retinal detachment on the same day to allow rapid surgery (Figures 4.10 and 4.11). Once the macula is detached, urgency varies with the duration of the loss of central vision. If the duration is short, less than 3 days, refer as an emergency to allow rapid surgery and reduce the injury to the foveal cones. If the duration is 3–7 days, refer promptly within a couple of days; see Table 4.3 (Figures 4.12 and 4.13).

- Chance of 20/40 or better after fovea off retinal detachment[18]

• 10 days or less:	71%
• 11 days to 6 weeks:	27%
• More than 6 weeks:	14%

Table 4.2 Position of retinal breaks

Variable	Ratio (%)
Break size small	42.4
Break size medium	59.4
Break size large	20.9
Supratemporal	68.7
Inferotemporal	32.3
Supranasal	40.3
Inferonasal	17.0
Supratemporally attached	5.2
Supratemporally detached	63.3
Inferotemporally attached	8.0
Inferotemporally detached	26.2
Supranasally attached	9.4
Supranasally detached	34.7
Inferonasally attached	7.4
Inferonasally detached	11.2
Anterior	24.9
Posterior	14.2
4–5 and 7–8 clock hours flat breaks	4.1
5–7 clock hours flat breaks	7.3
4–5 and 7–8 clock hour breaks in RRD	10.6
5–7 clock hour breaks in RRD	10.2

Source: Williamson, T. H. et al., Characteristics of rhegmatogenous retinal detachment and their relationship to success rates of surgery, *Retina*, 34, 7, 1421–7, 2014.

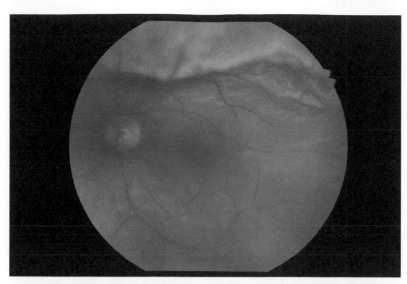

Figure 4.10 Retina is just lifting through the fovea.

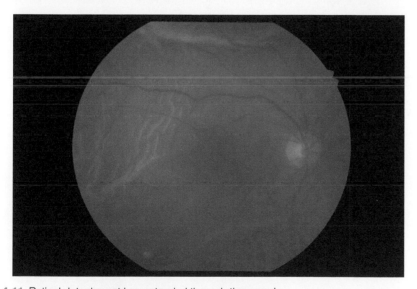

Figure 4.11 Retinal detachment has extended through the macula.

Table 4.3 Referral

Condition	Characteristics	Referral	Why?
RRD with PVD	Macula on	Immediate	Prevent macula from detaching
	Macula off for less than 1 week	1–2 days	Macula should recover fully
	Macula off for 1–2 weeks	3 days	Macula should recover well
	Macula off for 2–6 weeks	1 week	Macula will show moderate recovery
	Macula off for >6 weeks	2 weeks	Macula is unlikely to recover well
RRD without PVD		1 week	Slow progression

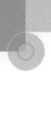

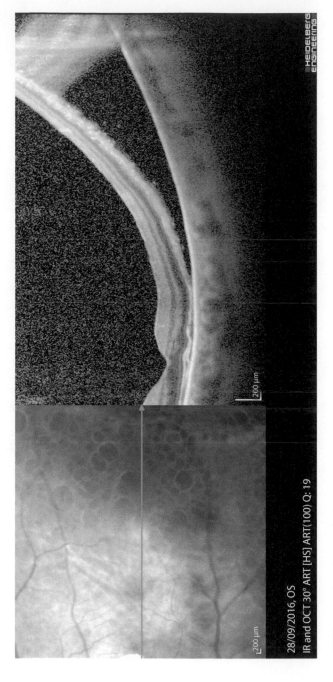

Figure 4.12 SRF is spreading close to the fovea.

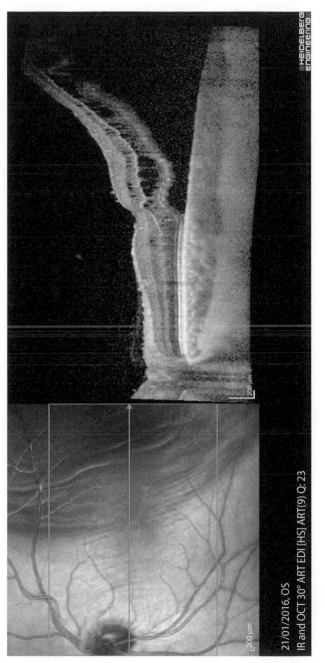

Figure 4.13 Optical coherence tomography (OCT) shows extension of the SRF under the fovea.

Visual recovery after surgery for RRD shows that high to moderate levels of visual acuity can be achieved in most patients with the following statistics:

- 27.1% achieving 20/20 or better
- 39.0% achieving 20/30 to 20/40
- 24.6% achieving 20/50 to 20/200

The primary success of surgery, PVR, presenting visual acuity and number of quadrants of RRD, is significantly associated with achieving vision of 20/30 or better.[19,20] Those patients whose retina is fixed with one operation have better visual results. PVR is the strongest risk factor for failure of surgery, and therefore, it is unsurprising that it was associated with reduced vision. Surgeons have been reassured by publications which show no difference in visual recovery in patients with foveal-off RRD and varying duration of symptoms in the first week[21–25] or first 10 days,[18] but more recent studies show reduced visual results for patients with 1–3-day duration and those with 4–7-day duration, in eyes without PVR.[26] There is one line of difference of visual recovery between patients with fovea on and 1 day of fovea off.

Macula-off retinal detachments are probably more likely to suffer subtle changes in vision such as distortion post-operatively; therefore, it is preferable to avoid the detachment of the fovea by performing surgery on 'macula-on' retinal detachment promptly, e.g. within 24 hours.[27] Autofluorescence studies however can show evidence of retinal macular shift even in macula-on retinal detachment post-operatively, indicating that there may be a shift of SRF into the macula even in these patients[28]; therefore, the situation is not entirely clear.

Chronic retinal detachments (e.g. when the vitreous is attached), in which there is slow accumulation of SRF, can be left longer before surgery. This requires careful identification of the type of retinal detachment presentation, which is associated with slow progression such as retinal dialysis and round holes.

By posturing a retinal break to the dependant portion of the eye, the accumulation of SRF can be reduced or even reversed while the patient is waiting for surgery.

- For a temporal hole in the left eye or a nasal hole in the right eye, the patient would be asked to lie with their left cheek down to the ground.
- For a nasal hole in the left eye or a temporal hole in the right eye, the patient would be asked to lie with their right cheek down to the ground.
- For a superior hole, the patient lies supine with no pillows and the foot of the bed raised.
- For inferior holes, sit the patient upright.

FLAT RETINAL BREAKS

RETINOPEXY

If a patient presents with a retinal break, which is at high risk of producing a retinal detach-ment (U tear, paravascular tear, operculated tear or dialysis), but has no SRF, then retinopexy is applied to prevent the accumulation of fluid underneath the neurosensory retina.[29] This can be applied as laser therapy around the break (usually in two rows around the circumference of the break) or by transscleral cryotherapy. Both methods produce damage to the neurosen-sory retina, the RPE, Bruch's layer and choroid. The scar formation seals the layers of the ret-ina together, preventing the fluid from passing through the hole and occurs in approximately 5–10 days (Figure 4.14).

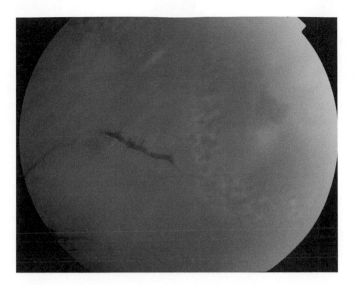

Figure 4.14 Tear has been surrounded by laser. There is some paravascular lattice in addition.

CRYOTHERAPY

Cryotherapy employs the Joule–Thomson effect, whereby the expansion of certain gases, such as nitrous oxide or carbon dioxide, results in a reduction in temperature. The gas is compressed and then released through a small hole in a cryotherapy instrument tip, causing a rapid expansion of the gas and reduction in the temperature. Cryotherapy has the advantage that it can be applied from the outside of the eye. The freeze damages the internal layers, causing scar formation.

It takes effect and has maximum adhesion in approximately 10 days but causes dispersion of retinal pigment epithelial cells into the vitreous giving an increased risk of PVR especially in the presence of U tears with curled edges or tears greater than 180°.[30]

LASER

Argon, diode or visible spectrum diode laser induce tissue injury and, therefore, scarring, from thermal burns on the tissues (photocoagulation). The laser should extend anteriorly around the tear or if not possible should extend to the ora serrata to prevent fluid ingress. Argon laser therapy can be applied either by a contact lens with a slit lamp or by indirect ophthalmoscopy with indentation. Maximum adhesion takes approximately 5 days and requires two rows of burns around a break for maximal adhesion.

RHEGMATOGENOUS RETINAL DETACHMENT

The definition of RRD is a retinal break with SRF. This may be as little as a small cuff of fluid or as much as total retinal detachment. Once the detachment has occurred, identification and closure of the retinal break or breaks is the primary aim of surgery. Once all the breaks are sealed, the retinal detachment should not return.

The attachment of a silastic explant to the sclera of the eye to create a dent in the sphere of the eye underneath the break or breaks allows the retina to reattach. This may occur because of relief of traction or because of an alteration in the fluid currents in the eye.

Alternatively, the vitreous is removed by pars plana vitrectomy (PPV). A long-acting gas bubble, such as sulphahexafluoride or perfluoropropane, is inserted into the vitreous cavity. The gas bubble contacts the rim of the break, preventing the passage of fluid through the break (tamponade). Thereafter, SRF will be reabsorbed by the RPE and the retina will flatten.

The gas bubble is only temporary until the retinal breaks are sealed. The indentation from an explant may gradually lessen with time. Retinopexy is applied to seal the tear and avoid the reaccumulation of the SRF.

The shortening on the retina produced by PVR may prevent retinal reattachment unless the fibrous membranes are surgically removed or the retina is cut to fit inside the eye (retinectomy). In this circumstance, silicone oil may be inserted into the vitreous cavity to provide long-term support (as opposed to short-term support of gas) to the retina allowing time for the PVR process to stop. Silicone oil in the vitreous cavity is associated with a number of complications including the following:

- Cataract
- Glaucoma
- Refractive changes
- Retinal toxicity

Although it is possible to perform most of these operations by vitrectomy alone, this may be inconvenient for the patient in that they will often develop a cataract requiring further surgery later. They may also be required to position their heads for 1–2 weeks and will have delayed visual recovery for 2–8 weeks depending on the gas used. A conventional procedure using an explant, on the other hand, does not produce cataract and requires no posturing in most circumstances. However, it requires opening of the conjunctiva and placement of a foreign body (the explant) onto the sclera.

Many surgeons will now treat most RRD with PVD by PPV, and those with attached vitreous are operated by explant procedure; however, there is wide a variation in methods worldwide.

PRINCIPLES OF SURGERY

The principles of surgery are as follows:

- Break closure
- Relief of traction
- Alteration of fluid currents
- Retinopexy[31]

PARS PLANA VITRECTOMY

PPV is becoming more popular for RRD repair because of the ease of application and good visualisation of the retina with wide-angle viewing systems. The examination of Medicare data for fees in the United States shows a 72% increase in the use of PPV for RRD and a 69% reduction in the use of scleral buckles from 1997 to 2007.[32] In addition, cataract can easily be dealt with per-operatively or post-operatively by phacoemulsification and posterior chamber lens implant (Figures 4.15 through 4.20).

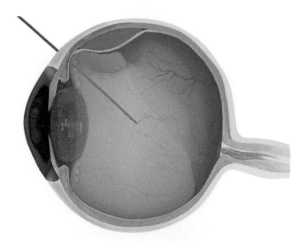

Figure 4.15 PPV is used to remove the vitreous to get access to the retinal detachment.

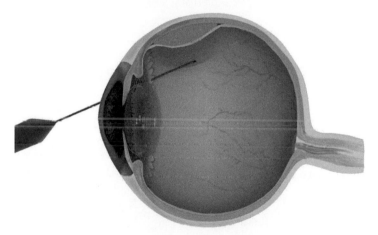

Figure 4.16 Surgeon can drain the fluid from the subretinal space through the retinal break to flatten the retina.

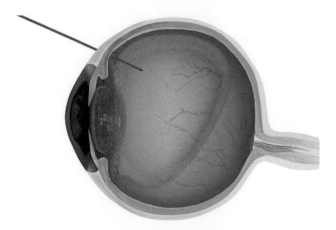

Figure 4.17 Gas bubble is inserted to hold the retina in place for a few weeks post-operatively.

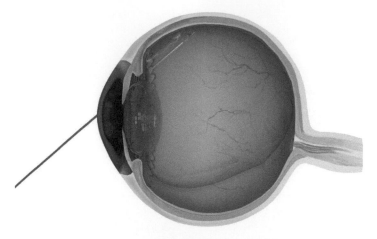

Figure 4.18 Laser burns are applied around the retinal break to seal off the retina around the break and prevent vitreous cavity fluid entering the subretinal space.

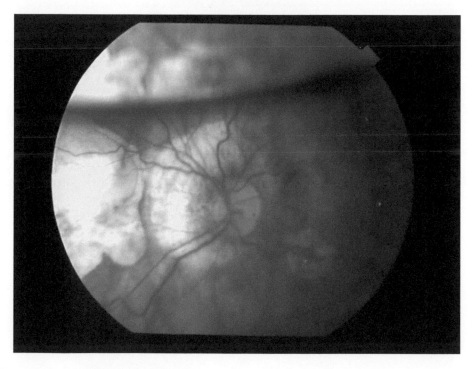

Figure 4.19 Gas bubble in a myopic eye.

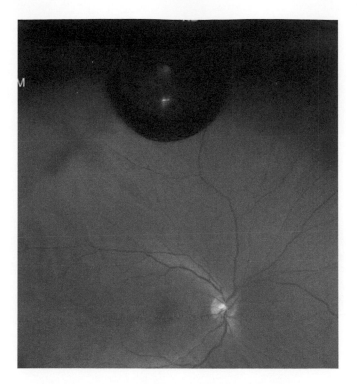

Figure 4.20 Small residual gas bubble in the vitreous cavity. Gas bubbles are used to hold the retina in place until retinopexy has sealed the retinal breaks. It absorbs spontaneously.

POSTURING

Some surgeons will ask the patient to position post-operatively to maximise the effect of the gas bubble. The patient does not need to posture if the breaks are above the horizontal meridian. Posturing can be employed for breaks inferior to three and nine o'clock. They would usually only posture for the first 7 days post-operatively.

- For a temporal hole in the left eye or a nasal hole in the right eye, the patient would be asked to lie with their right cheek down to the ground.
- For a nasal hole in the left eye or a temporal hole in the right eye, the patient would be asked to lie with their left cheek down to the ground.
- For an inferior hole, the patient lies supine (face up) with no pillows and the foot of the bed raised if possible.

NON-DRAIN PROCEDURE

The surgery for RRD evolved over the twentieth century from surgery with scleral buckling[33] to PPV and gas (Figures 4.21 and 4.22).[34] The non-drain retinal detachment procedure involves the placement of a silicone sponge underneath a retinal tear. The placement of the sponge is crucial to the success of the procedure, but it avoids the use of gas and had less risk of inducing cataract. It is often reserved for patients with vitreous-attached retinal detachment (Figures 4.23 through 4.26).

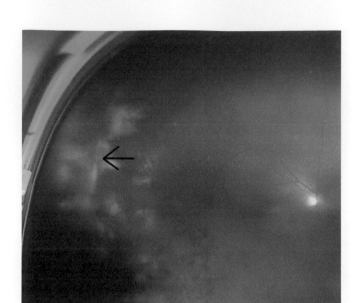

Figure 4.21 Scleral explant has been used to flatten a chronic retinal detachment.

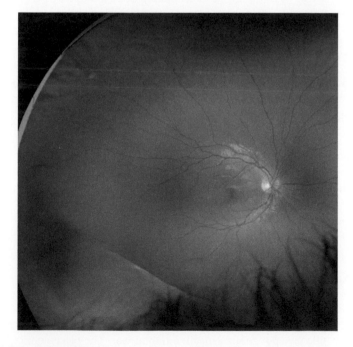

Figure 4.22 Inferior indentation of the retina from a scleral buckle.

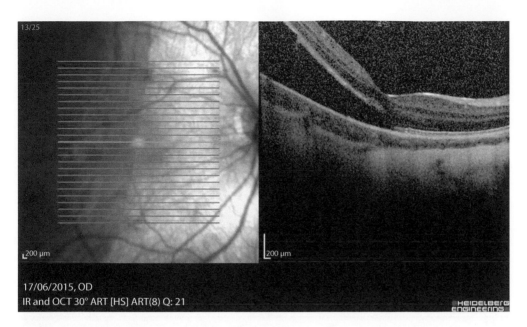

13/25

200 μm

200 μm

17/06/2015, OD
IR and OCT 30° ART [HS] ART(8) Q: 21

Figure 4.23 OCT of SRF spreading under the fovea.

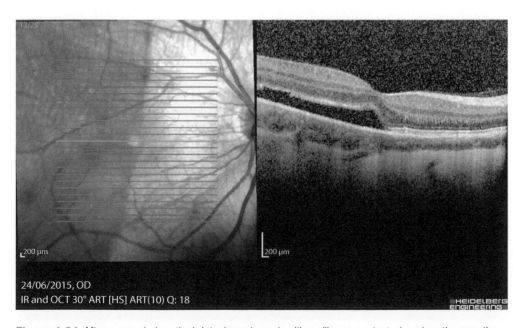

13/25

200 μm

200 μm

24/06/2015, OD
IR and OCT 30° ART [HS] ART(10) Q: 18

Figure 4.24 After a non-drain retinal detachment repair with a silicone explant placed on the eye, the SRF at the macula slowly reabsorbs over months.

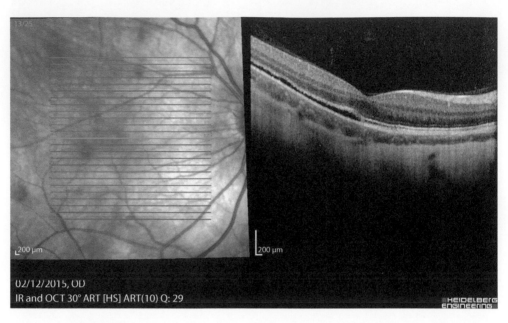

Figure 4.25 SRF reduces.

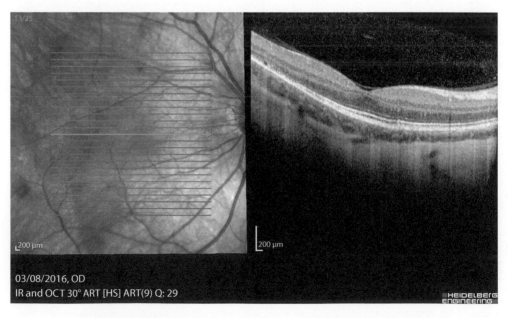

Figure 4.26 Finally, the retina is attached fully in this case with 20/25 vision.

PNEUMATIC RETINOPEXY

The successful reattachment of the retina can be achieved by the injection of gas and retinopexy without PPV,[35] especially with single superior breaks in the presence of a PVD. However, the success rates are lower than other methods, approximately 65% reattachment with one procedure,[36,37] and there is the risk of inducing new inferior retinal breaks.[38] Even in the best hands and with the selection of easy cases (one to two breaks), the success rate is 80%,[39] probably 10% less than the expected success rate from PPV on the same cases. In a recent analysis of Medicare insurance forms looking at individual patients rather than eyes, pneumatic retinopexy was twice as likely to be followed by further surgery (40%) than PPV or scleral buckling (20%) despite PPV being used for more complex cases but with PPV having twice the adverse complication rate (2%).[3]

SUCCESS RATES

Primary (flat retina after one operation) and secondary (flat retina after multiple operations) success rates depend in particular on the case mix of patients, rates of PVR at presentation and speed of access to surgery.

Primary:
- 81–92% in uncomplicated cases[40–46]
- 65–70% in high risk eyes or 75% when no break is found[41,47–51]

Secondary or final success rates should be approximately 95–97%,[52] but this drops in PVR and when no break is found.[53]

A visual outcome of 20/40 is achievable in most patients[41] and 83% of fovea on patients.[15] Visual outcome in foveal detachment is reduced to a 44% chance of 20/40 or better. Patients may describe metamorphopsia (change in image shape) after macula-off retinal detachment, and this may be accompanied by a reduction in stereo acuity.[27]

CAUSES OF FAILURE

Surgical capability will affect the success rate of such technical operations. Missing and therefore failing to treat breaks or new breaks will lead to redetachment in half of the failures. PVR is less predictable and controllable causing failure in the remainder.[54] In addition, severe complications of surgery must be added such as endophthalmitis and choroidal haemorrhage. Persistent thin areas of SRF have been described on OCT, occasionally affecting the macula, and thereby reducing visual acuity in buckling procedures.[55,56] Late macular breaks have been described in rare cases after scleral buckle.[57] Late redetachments over 1 year can occur in approximately 2%.[58] The cause is usually from new break formation, although old breaks can reopen.

PROLIFERATIVE VITREORETINOPATHY

INTRODUCTION

There are two reasons that delay in referral of retinal detachments is problematic. The first is the detrimental effect on vision when the retinal receptors have been detached for a prolonged period, and the second is the onset of PVR. This is a scarring process, which produces ERM in RRD. It occurs in RRDs, which have been present for weeks or months. At presentation, the rate of PVR in all patients with RRD often varies with the ease of access to healthcare. Prompt surgery reduces PVR rates to 5%; however, where there is delay, PVR rates are much higher, e.g. 53% in parts of South America[59] and 17.5% in East Africa.[60] Failure of surgery increases the risk of post-operative PVR, e.g. 5% of RRDs with U tears, 18% with paravascular tears and 25% of giant retinal tears.[30]

PVR development is inconsistent with some eyes, producing a response after a short duration and others with chronic detachment remaining free from proliferation. Other conditions with retinal detachment are at high risk of PVR such as severe ocular trauma and some inflammatory conditions, e.g. acute retinal necrosis.

PATHOGENESIS

The retinal pigment epithelial cell is the main source of the proliferation.[61] These cells disperse into the vitreous cavity through a retinal break. They change into scar tissue producing cells, which produce collagen. As with any scar tissue, contraction occurs.

Note: Contraction of a wound on a planar surface closes the wound by drawing the wound edges together. However, inside the surface of a sphere such as the eye, the contraction tends to drag tissue (in this case, the neurosensory retina) into the centre of the sphere, exacerbating the retinal detachment process.

In addition, the retina itself becomes short and stiff and more difficult to reattach to the inner surface of the posterior segment of the eye.

CLINICAL FEATURES

INTRODUCTION

PVR is characterised by shortening, stiffening and folding of the retina progressing to a funnel retinal detachment, which is immobile. Fibrosis can be seen on the inner and outer surfaces of the retina. PVR opens up existing tears, creates new tears and induces retinal detachment even when no open tears are found.[62] Pre-operative PVR increases the risk of developing severe post-operative PVR.[63]

GRADING

PVR is graded as follows (Figure 4.27) (Table 4.4)[64]:

- A: Clumping of retinal pigment epithelial cells and stiffening of the vitreous.
- B: Partial-thickness folding of the inner retina
- C: Full-thickness fixed folding of the retina, commencing as localised star folds and progressing to an open funnel formation and then a closed funnel in the final stages. C PVR is quantified by locating the area of folding either anterior (A) or posterior (P) to the equator and by indicating the number of clock hours of retina involved (1–12).

Occasionally, the proliferation is predominantly subretinal,[65] producing fibrous strands which elevate the retina, like the guy ropes of a tent, or even 'purse string' the retina around the optic disc (Figure 4.28).

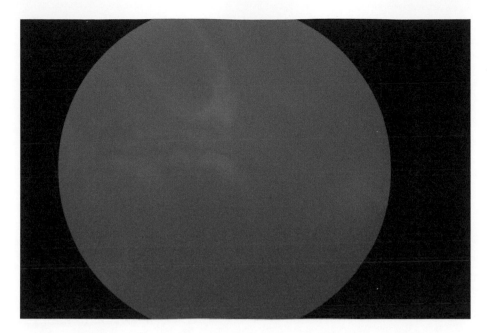

Figure 4.27 Membrane on the surface of the retina causes a 'star fold' of the retina in early PVR.

Table 4.4 Grading PVR

Grading	
A	Vitreous haze, pigment clumps, pigment clusters on inferior retina
B	Inner retinal wrinkling, retinal stiffness, rolled break edges, vitreous stiffness
CP 1–12	Full-thickness retinal folds or subretinal strands posterior to the equator (described as 1–12 clock hours of involvement)
CA 1–12	Full-thickness retinal folds or subretinal strands anterior to the equator (described as 1–12 clock hours of involvement), anterior displacement, condensed vitreous strands

Descriptive terms		
Type	**Usual location**	**Features**
Focal	Posterior	Star folds in the retina
Diffuse	Posterior	Confluent retinal folding
Subretinal	Posterior	Fibrous strands, linear and purse string around the optic disc
		Fibrous sheets
Circumferential	Anterior	Contraction of the retina inwards at the posterior edge of the vitreous base
Anterior displacement	Anterior	Anterior traction on the retina at the vitreous base; ciliary body detachment and epiciliary membrane; iris retraction

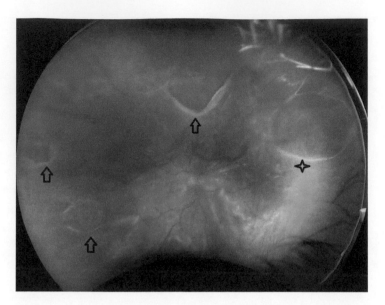

Figure 4.28 Chronic total RRD with retinal tears (*arrows*), a retinal cyst (*star*) and B PVR grade.

RISK OF PVR

PVR is more likely in the following cases:

- RRD for a prolonged period[59]
- Choroidal detachment[66]
- Previous surgery or cryotherapy[67]
- Pre-existing PVR
- Aphakia
- VH may increase the risk of PVR[68]
- Vascular abnormalities such as retina telangiectasia or angiomas
- Uveitis
- Trauma

SURGERY

RELIEVING RETINECTOMY

PVR requires extra surgical intervention (Figure 4.29). Often, the patient will require multiple operations over a prolonged period to flatten the retina. In many cases, silicone oil insertion is required. The complications of silicone oil are many, and therefore, it is preferable not to use this agent if possible. The stiff short retina may need to be cut to make it fit into the inner surface of the sphere. Some surgeons will use bands made of silicone to change the shape of the eye to help the retina settle.

SUCCESS RATES

The aim for these cases is to achieve reattached retina with silicone oil removed. Success rates are usually low in patients with PVR with single operations, approximately 62–65%[69–72] or even multiple operations 68–84%.[70,73,74] The success is poorer if silicone oil removal is a requirement

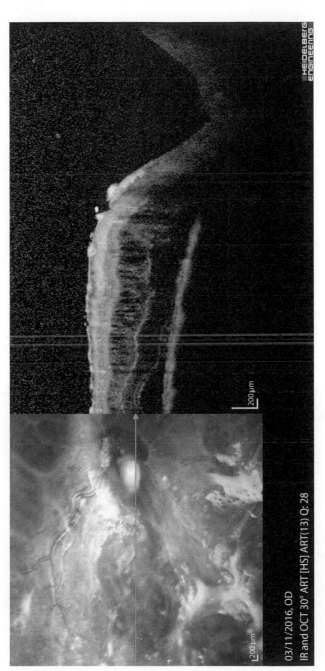

03/11/2016, OD

IR and OCT 30° ART [HS] ART(13) Q: 28

Figure 4.29 Severe fibrosis on the retina from PVR.

of success, e.g. 51–81%.[75,76] Patients who achieve a reattached retina with the one operation have significantly better visual outcomes.[77] The visual outcome is a 24–45% chance of 20/200 vision or better.[73,78] In addition, these patients often have distortion of the vision. There is a risk that the poor vision can interfere with the vision in the patient binocularly.

There is a risk of sight threatening complications in the other eye of these patients (50%), which helps justify the surgery in the eye despite poor success rates.[79]

It is best to remove the oil because of the attendant complications of glaucoma, band keratopathy and central visual loss.

The cause of failure of surgery is usually further PVR formation[80] with reoperations required at 2 months (Figures 4.30 through 4.32).

SURGERY FOR REDETACHMENT

Despite the surgeon's greatest efforts, the redetachment of the retina occurs at rates of 10–15%. The rate of redetachment is closely linked to the PVR rate at presentation with higher rates with more PVR.

Causes of redetachment are as follows:

- *PVR:* The surgery stimulates the PVR to progress, overcoming the effects of internal tamponade and reopening retinal breaks causing RRD.
  - Be aware of the presence of PVR at presentation; use longer-acting gases or silicone oil; restrict the use of cryotherapy
- *Missed retinal breaks:* Tiny retinal breaks may be missed during the first surgery; usually, these are easier to see at the second operation because slight contraction of the remaining vitreous base causes the breaks to open up slightly.

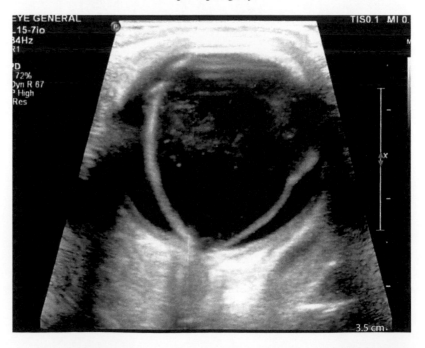

Figure 4.30 Ultrasound of a retinal detachment with PVR shows a stiff and shortened retina.

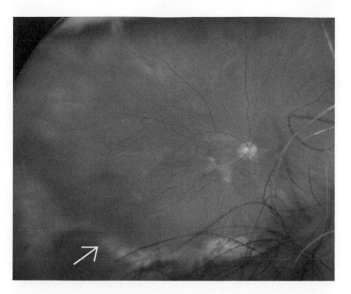

Figure 4.31 PVR shortens the retina. This prevents the reposition of the retina onto the inside of the sphere of the eye. The retina may need to be cut usually inferiorly to allow the retina to open out onto the inner surface of the eye. This is called a retinectomy and can be seen as an edge of retina with laser scars.

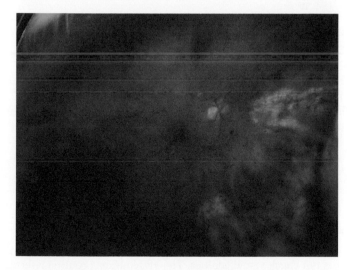

Figure 4.32 Inferior retinectomy with radial cuts has been used to reattach this retinal detachment.

- *New retinal breaks:* Occasionally, larger breaks appear that are unlikely to be missed from the first operation; these may be produced from problems at the sclerotomies (entry site breaks) or secondary to PVR.
- *PVR and missed/new breaks:* Often, the two accompany each other, and it is not possible to say with certainty which is the cause of the redetachment. However, if a break is found which was not treated at the first operation by retinopexy, it was probably missed or created at the first surgery and is therefore the cause of the redetachment; the PVR is secondary. This emphasises the importance of seeing and treating all pathology at the first operation and, therefore, the need for a technically competent surgeon.

SECONDARY MACULAR HOLES

Macular holes can be found associated with RRD pre-operatively and can spontaneously close after surgery without any additional procedures.[81] Holes that develop after surgery can occur in 1% of patients usually after scleral buckle of macular off RRD.[57] Those that do not close spontaneously can be treated by PPV and gas as for idiopathic macular holes. Posterior breaks have been described in the post-operative period around the arcades after PPV, which can be treated by laser retinopexy, although it is possible that no treatment is required.[82]

DETACHMENT WITH CHOROIDAL EFFUSIONS

If the retina detaches into the pars ciliaris, hypotony occurs and choroidal effusions may form. These can be drained early in the PPV through the sclerotomies using positive pressure from the infusion (take care when inserting the infusion that the tip has penetrated in to the vitreous cavity).[83,84] The fluid is often greenish in colour. Once the suprachoroidal fluid has drained, the RRD can be managed by the usual processes, although some advocate the use of silicone oil because these patients probably have an increased risk of PVR.[85] Others suggest pre-operative systemic steroid therapy.[86] Note that very rarely, a sequence of events is seen whereby the following occur (Table 4.3):

1. A break causes RRD.
2. RRD causes hypotony.
3. Hypotony causes effusions.
4. Effusions indent onto the retinal break.
5. The RRD subsides.
6. Leaving a flat retinal break on an apparently spontaneous choroidal effusion, laser the break and wait for the effusions to settle.

MEDICOLEGAL CASES

CASE 1

An elderly man with a complex medical history and with 6 months of reduced vision is assessed by an FP, who does not check visual acuities. The FP requests a routine referral to a hospital. One month later, the patient attends an optometrist, who then diagnoses severe cataracts on the basis of a poor red reflex in each eye. There is reduction in vision in both eyes. The optometrist finds the patient uncooperative and is unable to obtain IOP measurements. A decision is taken not to dilate the patient's pupils as a result. A referral is instigated to the FP, indicating a need for urgent referral but with a diagnosis of cataract. This is confusing to other healthcare professionals in reference to the urgency of referral. Eventually, the patient attends ophthalmology after a delay of 3 months and is found to have bilateral total retinal detachments with severe proliferative retinopathy and very poor vision. A decision not to operate was made by the attending surgeon. The negligent assessments by both the FP and optometrist lead to a poorer outcome in this case.

ERRORS

- Poor assessment of history
- FP did not check vision
- Optometrist demonstrated inadequate skills
- No rapid referral in a situation of doubt

Take-home message: Be sure you have the competency to make a diagnosis; if not, make sure that someone who has those competencies sees the patient.

CASE 2

A young myopic patient experiences a drop in vision in one eye. He attends an eye casualty but is turned away by a triage nurse without an examination. A week later, he attends an FP, who does not check the vision or examine the eye. Two weeks later, another FP refers the patient urgently to the hospital. The patient is seen at the hospital ophthalmology service 1 month after the initial presentation. The retina is detached with round holes and has an attached vitreous. The fovea is detached. Although the retina is successfully reattached by surgery, the vision is reduced.

ERRORS

- No examination by the nurse
- No vision check by the FP
- Slow referral by the FP
- Slow referral procedure performed

Take-home message: Do a visual acuity test.

CASE 3

A patient had bilateral cataract extractions with good visual results. Ten years later, the patient attends an FP, complaining of reduced vision in one eye. The vision has been reduced for a few days, associated with flashing lights. The FP finds a reduced red reflex in the eye and diagnoses a thickened posterior capsule. The FP sends a referral for a routine appointment for yttrium aluminium garnet capsulotomy.

The referral letter is delayed within the administration system of the hospital. The patient attends the hospital service after some months. The patient is found to have a total retinal detachment with PVR. Surgery was unsuccessful in reattaching the retina.

ERRORS

- The symptoms of flashes in the vision do not fit the diagnosis of posterior capsule opacity and are a symptom of posterior vitreous detachment.
- Although a reduced red reflex could occur with a very severe posterior capsule thickening, the clinical sign should suggest a retinal pathology.
- Again, the vision should be checked which would be worse with retinal detachment than PC thickening.

REFERENCES

1. Saidkasimova, S., Mitry, D., Singh, J. et al. Retinal detachment in Scotland is associated with affluence. *Br J Ophthalmol* 2009;93(12):1591–4.
2. Williamson, T. H., Lee, E. J. and Shunmugam, M. Characteristics of rhegmatogenous retinal detachment and their relationship to success rates of surgery. *Retina* 2014;34(7):1421–7.
3. Day, S., Grossman, D. S., Mruthyunjaya, P. et al. One-year outcomes after retinal detachment surgery among medicare beneficiaries. *Am J Ophthalmol* 2010;150(3):338–45.
4. Ung, T., Comer, M. B., Ang, A. J. et al. Clinical features and surgical management of retinal detachment secondary to round retinal holes. *Eye* 2004.
5. Williams, K. M., Dogramaci, M. and Williamson, T. H. Retrospective study of rhegmatogenous retinal detachments secondary to round retinal holes. *Eur J Ophthalmol* 2012;22(4):635–40.
6. Marcus, D. F. and Aaberg, T. M. Intraretinal macrocysts in retinal detachment. *Arch Ophthalmol* 1979;97(7):1273–5.
7. Ahmed, I., McDonald, H. R., Schatz, H. et al. Crystalline retinopathy associated with chronic retinal detachment. *Arch Ophthalmol* 1998;116(11):1449–53.
8. Laatikainen, L. and Tolppanen, E. M. Characteristics of rhegmatogenous retinal detachment. *Acta Ophthalmol (Copenh)* 1985;63(2):146–54.
9. Krohn, J. and Seland, J. H. Simultaneous, bilateral rhegmatogenous retinal detachment. *Acta Ophthalmol Scand* 2000;78(3):354–8.
10. Gonzales, C. R., Gupta, A., Schwartz, S. D. and Kreiger, A. E. The fellow eye of patients with rhegmatogenous retinal detachment. *Ophthalmology* 2004;111(3):518–21.
11. Netland, P. A., Mukai, S. and Covington, H. I. Elevated intraocular pressure secondary to rhegmatogenous retinal detachment. *Surv Ophthalmol* 1994;39(3):234–40.
12. Schwartz, A. Chronic open-angle glaucoma secondary to rhegmatogenous retinal detachment. *Trans Am Ophthalmol Soc* 1972;70:178–89.
13. Tanaka, S., Ideta, H., Yonemoto, J. et al. Neovascularization of the iris in rhegmatogenous retinal detachment. *Am J Ophthalmol* 1991;112(6):632–4.
14. Shafer, D. M., Stratford, D. P., Schepens, C. L. and Regan, C. J. D. Binocular indirect opthalmoscopy. In *Controversial Aspects of the Management of the Retinal Detachment*. London: J & A Churchill, 2005.
15. Ho, S. F., Fitt, A., Frimpong-Ansah, K. and Benson, M. T. The management of primary rhegmatogenous retinal detachment not involving the fovea. *Eye (Lond)* 2006;20(9):1049–53.
16. Hammer, M. E., Burch, T. G. and Rinder, D. Viscosity of subretinal fluid and its clinical correlations. *Retina* 1986;6(4):234–8.
17. Lincoff, H. and Gieser, R. Finding the retinal hole. *Arch Ophthalmol* 1971;85(5):565–9.
18. Hassan, T. S., Sarrafizadeh, R., Ruby, A. J. et al. The effect of duration of macular detachment on results after the scleral buckle repair of primary, macula-off retinal detachments. *Ophthalmology* 2002;109(1):146–52.
19. Salicone, A., Smiddy, W. E., Venkatraman, A. and Feuer, W. Visual recovery after scleral buckling procedure for retinal detachment. *Ophthalmology* 2006;113(10):1734–42.
20. Oshima, Y., Yamanishi, S., Sawa, M. et al. Two-year follow-up study comparing primary vitrectomy with scleral buckling for macula-off rhegmatogenous retinal detachment. *Jpn J Ophthalmol* 2000;44(5):538–49.

21. Ross, W., Lavina, A., Russell, M. and Maberley, D. The correlation between height of macular detachment and visual outcome in macula-off retinal detachments of ≤7 days' duration. *Ophthalmology* 2005;112(7):1213–7.

22. Ross, W. H. Visual recovery after macula-off retinal detachment. *Eye* 2002;16(4):440–6.

23. Ross, W. H. and Kozy, D. W. Visual recovery in macula-off rhegmatogenous retinal detachments. *Ophthalmology* 1998;105(11):2149–53.

24. Ross, W. H. and Stockl, F. A. Visual recovery after retinal detachment. *Curr Opin Ophthalmol* 2000;11(3):191–4.

25. Diederen, R. M., La Heij, E. C., Kessels, A. G. et al. Scleral buckling surgery after macula-off retinal detachment: Worse visual outcome after more than 6 days. *Ophthalmology* 2007;114(4):705–9.

26. Williamson, T. H., Shunmugam, M., Rodrigues, I. et al. Characteristics of rhegmatogenous retinal detachment and their relationship to visual outcome. *Eye (Lond)* 2013;27(9):1063–9.

27. Ugarte, M. and Williamson, T. H. Horizontal and vertical micropsia following macula-off rhegmatogenous retinal-detachment surgical repair. *Graefes Arch Clin Exp Ophthalmol* 2006;244(11):1545–8.

28. Lee, E., Williamson, T. H., Hysi, P. et al. Macular displacement following rhegmatogenous retinal detachment repair. *Br J Ophthalmol* 2013;97(10):1297–302.

29. Gonin, J. The treatment of detached retina by searing the retinal tears. *Arch Ophthalmol* 1930;4:621–3.

30. Bonnet, M., Fleury, J., Guenoun, S. et al. Cryopexy in primary rhegmatogenous retinal detachment: A risk factor for postoperative proliferative vitreoretinopathy? *Graefes Arch Clin Exp Ophthalmol* 1996;234(12):739–43.

31. Custodis, E. Beobachtungen bei der diathermischen Behandlung der Netzhautatablosung und ein Minweis zur Therapie der Operation der Netzhautablosung. *Ber Dtsch Opthalmol Ges* 1952(57):227–9.

32. Ramulu, P. Y., Do, D. V., Corcoran, K. J. et al. Use of retinal procedures in Medicare beneficiaries from 1997 to 2007. *Arch Ophthalmol* 2010;128(10):1335–40.

33. Custodis, E. Scleral prebuckling with plastic plombage. *Bibl Ophthalmol* 1965;65:140–3.

34. Machemer, R., Parel, J. M. and Norton, E. W. Vitrectomy: A pars plana approach. Technical improvements and further results. *Trans Am Acad Ophthalmol Otolaryngol* 1972;76(2):462–6.

35. Hilton, G. F. and Grizzard, W. S. Pneumatic retinopexy. A two-step outpatient operation without conjunctival incision. *Ophthalmology* 1986;93(5):626–41.

36. McAllister, I. L., Meyers, S. M., Zegarra, H. et al. Comparison of pneumatic retinopexy with alternative surgical techniques. *Ophthalmology* 1988;95(7):877–83.

37. Han, D. P., Mohsin, N. C., Guse, C. E. et al. Comparison of pneumatic retinopexy and scleral buckling in the management of primary rhegmatogenous retinal detachment. Southern Wisconsin Pneumatic Retinopexy Study Group. *Am J Ophthalmol* 1998;126(5):658–68.

38. Poliner, L. S., Grand, M. G. Schoch, L. H. et al. New retinal detachment after pneumatic retinopexy. *Ophthalmology* 1987;94(4):315–8.

39. Mudvari, S. S., Ravage, Z. B. and Rezaci, K. A. Retinal detachment after primary pneumatic retinopexy. *Retina* 2009;29(10):1474–8.

40. Ah-Fat, F. G., Sharma, M. C., Majid, M. A. et al. Trends in vitreoretinal surgery at a tertiary referral centre: 1987 to 1996. *Br J Ophthalmol* 1999;83(4):396–8.

41. Campo, R.V., Sipperley, J.O., Sneed, S. R. et al. Pars plana vitrectomy without scleral buckle for pseudophakic retinal detachments. *Ophthalmology* 1999;106(9):1811–5.
42. Girard, P. and Karpouzas, I. Pseudophakic retinal detachment: Anatomic and visual results. *Graefes Arch Clin Exp Ophthalmol* 1995;233(6):324–30.
43. La Heij, E. C., Derhaag, P. F. and Hendrikse, F. Results of scleral buckling operations in primary rhegmatogenous retinal detachment. *Doc Ophthalmol* 2000;100(1):17–25.
44. Oshima, Y., Emi, K., Motokura, M. and Yamanishi, S. Survey of surgical indications and results of primary pars plana vitrectomy for rhegmatogenous retinal detachments. *Jpn J Ophthalmol* 1999;43(2):120–6.
45. Thompson, J. A., Snead, M. P., Billington, B. M. et al. National audit of the outcome of primary surgery for rhegmatogenous retinal detachment. II. Clinical outcomes. *Eye* 2002;16(6):771–7.
46. Minihan, M., Tanner, V. and Williamson, T. H. Primary rhegmatogenous retinal detachment: 20 years of change. *Br J Ophthalmol* 2001;85(5):546–8.
47. Hakin, K. N., Lavin, M. J. and Leaver, P. K. Primary vitrectomy for rhegmatogenous retinal detachment. *Graefes Arch Clin Exp Ophthalmol* 1993;231(6):344–6.
48. Heimann, H., Bornfeld, N., Friedrichs, W. et al. Primary vitrectomy without scleral buckling for rhegmatogenous retinal detachment. *Graefes Arch Clin Exp Ophthalmol* 1996;234(9):561–8.
49. Schmidt, J.C., Rodrigues, E. B., Hoerle, S. et al. Primary vitrectomy in complicated rhegmatogenous retinal detachment – A survey of 205 eyes. *Ophthalmologica* 2003;217(6):387–92.
50. Tewari, H. K., Kedar, S., Kumar, A. et al. Comparison of scleral buckling with combined scleral buckling and pars plana vitrectomy in the management of rhegmatogenous retinal detachment with unseen retinal breaks. *Clin Experiment Ophthalmol* 2003;31(5):403–7.
51. Wong, D., Billington, B. M. and Chignell, A. H. Pars plana vitrectomy for retinal detachment with unseen retinal holes. *Graefes Arch Clin Exp Ophthalmol* 1987;225(4):269–71.
52. Doyle, E., Herbert, E. N., Bunce, C. et al. How effective is macula-off retinal detachment surgery: Might good outcome be predicted? *Eye* 2007;21(4):534–40.
53. Salicone, A., Smiddy, W. E., Venkatraman, A. and Feuer, W. Management of retinal detachment when no break is found. *Ophthalmology* 2006;113(3):398–403.
54. Richardson, E. C., Verma, S., Green, W. T. et al. Primary vitrectomy for rhegmatogenous retinal detachment: An analysis of failure. *Eur J Ophthalmol* 2000;10(2):160–6.
55. Baba, T., Hirose, A., Moriyama, M. and Mochizuki, M. Tomographic image and visual recovery of acute macula-off rhegmatogenous retinal detachment. *Graefes Arch Clin Exp Ophthalmol* 2004;242(7):576–81.
56. Wolfensberger, T. J. and Gonvers, M. Optical coherence tomography in the evaluation of incomplete visual acuity recovery after macula-off retinal detachments. *Graefes Arch Clin Exp Ophthalmol* 2002;240(2):85–9.
57. Moshfeghi, A. A., Salam, G. A., Deramo, V. A. et al. Management of macular holes that develop after retinal detachment repair. *Am J Ophthalmol* 2003;136(5):895–9.
58. Foster, R. E. and Meyers, S. M. Recurrent retinal detachment more than 1 year after reattachment. *Ophthalmology* 2002;109(10):1821–7.
59. Tseng, W., Cortez, R. T., Ramirez, G. et al. Prevalence and risk factors for proliferative vitreoretinopathy in eyes with rhegmatogenous retinal detachment but no previous vitreoretinal surgery. *Am J Ophthalmol* 2004;137(6):1105–15.

60. Yorston, D. B., Wood, M. L. and Gilbert, C. Retinal detachment in East Africa. *Ophthalmology* 2002;109(12):2279–83.

61. Glaser, B. M., Cardin, A. and Biscoe, B. Proliferative vitreoretinopathy. The mechanism of development of vitreoretinal traction. *Ophthalmology* 1987;94(4):327–32.

62. Moisseiev, J. and Glaser, B. M. New and previously unidentified retinal breaks in eyes with recurrent retinal detachment with proliferative vitreoretinopathy. *Arch Ophthalmol* 1989;107(8):1152–4.

63. Kon, C. H., Asaria, R. H., Occleston, N. L. et al. Risk factors for proliferative vitreoretinopathy after primary vitrectomy: A prospective study. *Br J Ophthalmol* 2000;84(5):506–11.

64. Machemer, R., Aaberg, T. M, Freeman, H. M. et al. An updated classification of retinal detachment with proliferative vitreoretinopathy. *Am J Ophthalmol* 1991;112(2):159–65.

65. Lewis, H., Aaberg, T. M., Abrams, G. W. et al. Subretinal membranes in proliferative vitreoretinopathy. *Ophthalmology* 1989;96(9):1403–14.

66. Cowley, M., Conway, B. P., Campochiaro, P. A. et al. Clinical risk factors for proliferative vitreoretinopathy. *Arch Ophthalmol* 1989;107(8):1147–51.

67. Glaser, B. M., Vidaurri-Leal, J., Michels, R. G. and Campochiaro, P. A. Cryotherapy during surgery for giant retinal tears and intravitreal dispersion of viable retinal pigment epithelial cells. *Ophthalmology* 1993;100(4):466–70.

68. Duquesne, N., Bonnet, M. and Adeleine, P. Preoperative vitreous hemorrhage associated with rhegmatogenous retinal detachment: A risk factor for postoperative proliferative vitreoretinopathy? *Graefes Arch Clin Exp Ophthalmol* 1996;234(11):677–82.

69. Stolba, U., Binder, S., Velikay, M. et al. Use of perfluorocarbon liquids in proliferative vitreoretinopathy: Results and complications. *Br J Ophthalmol* 1995;79(12):1106–10.

70. Han, D. P., Rychwalski, P. J., Mieler, W. F. and Abrams, G. W. Management of complex retinal detachment with combined relaxing retinotomy and intravitreal perfluoro-n-octane injection. *Am J Ophthalmol* 1994;118(1):24–32.

71. Fisher, Y. L., Shakin, J. L., Slakter, J. S. et al. Perfluoropropane gas, modified panretinal photocoagulation, and vitrectomy in the management of severe proliferative vitreoretinopathy. *Arch Ophthalmol* 1988;106(9):1255–60.

72. Cox, M. S., Trese, M. T. and Murphy, P. L. Silicone oil for advanced proliferative vitreoretinopathy. *Ophthalmology* 1986;93(5):646–50.

73. Scott, I. U., Flynn, H. W. Jr., Murray, T. G. and Feuer, W. J. Outcomes of surgery for retinal detachment associated with proliferative vitreoretinopathy using perfluoro-n-octane: A multicentre study. *Am J Ophthalmol* 2003;136(3):454–63.

74. Iverson, D. A., Ward, T. G. and Blumenkranz, M. S. Indications and results of relaxing retinotomy. *Ophthalmology* 1990;97(10):1298–304.

75. Charteris, D. G., Aylward, G. W., Wong, D. et al. A randomized controlled trial of combined 5–fluorouracil and low-molecular-weight heparin in management of established proliferative vitreoretinopathy. *Ophthalmology* 2004;111(12):2240–5.

76. Lam, R. F., Cheung, B.T., Yuen, C. Y. et al. Retinal redetachment after silicone oil removal in proliferative vitreoretinopathy: A prognostic factor analysis. *Am J Ophthalmol* 2008;145(3):527–33.

77. Scott, I. U., Flynn, H. W., Lai, M. et al. First operation anatomic success and other predictors of postoperative vision after complex retinal detachment repair with vitrectomy and silicone oil tamponade. *Am J Ophthalmol* 2000;130(6):745–50.

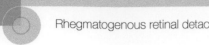
78. Vitrectomy with silicone oil or perfluoropropane gas in eyes with severe proliferative vitreoretinopathy: Results of a randomized clinical trial. Silicone Study Report 2. *Arch Ophthalmol* 1992;110(6):780–92.
79. Schwartz, S. D. and Kreiger, A. E. Proliferative vitreoretinopathy: A natural history of the fellow eye. *Ophthalmology* 1998;105(5):785–8.
80. Lewis, H. and Aaberg, T. M. Causes of failure after repeat vitreoretinal surgery for recurrent proliferative vitreoretinopathy. *Am J Ophthalmol* 1991;111(1):15–9.
81. Riordan-Eva, P. and Chignell, A. H. Full thickness macular breaks in rhegmatogenous retinal detachment with peripheral retinal breaks. *Br J Ophthalmol* 1992;76(6):346–8.
82. Okada, K., Sakata, H., Mizote, H. et al. Postoperative posterior retinal holes after pars plana vitrectomy for primary retinal detachment. *Retina* 1997;17(2):99–104.
83. Ghoraba, H. H. Primary vitrectomy for the management of rhegmatogenous retinal detachment associated with choroidal detachment. *Graefes Arch Clin Exp Ophthalmol* 2001;239(10):733–6.
84. Yang, C. M. Pars plana vitrectomy in the treatment of combined rhegmatogenous retinal detachment and choroidal detachment in aphakic or pseudophakic patients. *Ophthalmic Surg Lasers* 1997;28(4):288–93.
85. Loo, A., Fitt, A. W., Ramchandani, M. and Kirkby, G. R. Pars plana vitrectomy with silicone oil in the management of combined rhegmatogenous retinal and choroidal detachment. *Eye* 2001;15(Pt 5):612–5.
86. Sharma, T., Gopal, L. and Badrinath, S. S. Primary vitrectomy for rhegmatogenous retinal detachment associated with choroidal detachment. *Ophthalmology* 1998;105(12):2282–5.

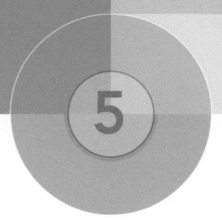

Different presentations of rhegmatogenous retinal detachments

5

AGE-RELATED RRD FROM PVD

The most common RRD is caused by an age-related PVD (Table 5.1).

PPV and gas with latter phacoemulsification cataract extraction and intraocular lens treat these. Scleral buckling procedures can also be applied. The description in the previous chapter is based on this common type of RRD (Figure 5.1).

ATROPHIC HOLE RRD WITH ATTACHED VITREOUS

Young myopic patients in the 20–40-year age group may present with a chronic RRD usually inferior and can be treated by non-drain surgery as described in the previous chapter (Table 5.2). Females comprise 64%, and 83% are myopic.[1] Abnormalities in the fellow eyes are common in 63%, with bilateral RRD in 12%.[2,3] These patients can go on to develop PVD with RRD from U tears in later life.

The slow progression of retinal detachment means that most cases can be referred over a few days. If you are confident of signs of chronicity, e.g. pigment demarcation of the edge of the RRD, then even slower referral can be made. If the fovea has just detached, it is worth getting the patient seen soon to determine how quickly the fovea needs to be reattached to improve results (often, it takes a while for the patient to notice the central vision loss however) (Figure 5.2).

PSEUDOPHAKIC RRD

Cataract surgery has evolved rapidly in the last 40 years with progression from intracapsular surgery and aphakia, to extracapsular surgery, to phacoemulsification and pseudophakia post-operatively. This has led to a reduction in complications and an improvement in the standard of surgery and post-operative outcome for cataract surgery worldwide. The causal relationship between cataract surgery and RRD is only partially defined from data from Medicare and other insurance information,[4–6] Scandinavian public health data[7,8] and large population-based studies such as the Rochester Study.[9,10] These suggest that there remains an increased risk of retinal detachment associated with cataract operations.

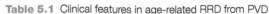

Table 5.1 Clinical features in age-related RRD from PVD

Sex	Males > females
Age	>40 years
Refraction	All refractions but more common in myopia
Bilateral	5%[2]
Fellow eye at presentation	5%
Onset	Rapid
Vitreous	Detached
Retinal break type	U tears, operculated breaks
Retinal break size	Variable
Mean number of breaks	2.5
Multiple breaks: >1	56%
Retinal break position	All quadrants but temporal > nasal and superior > inferior
Fovea off	55%
PVR	Preretinal A, B and C
Surgery	PPV and gas

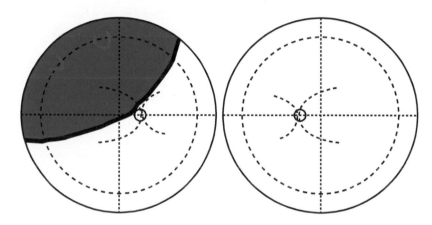

Figure 5.1 Most common position for a U-shaped retinal break is superotemporal, which leads to a rapidly progressive bullous retinal detachment. By convention, retinal detachments are blue and breaks in the retina red.

- The 4-year incidence of retinal detachment after all cataract extractions has been described as 1.17%
- Increasing with vitreous loss to 4.9%
- Reduced in phacoemulsification to 0.4%[11]

This is regarded as higher than would be expected in the normal population. Approximately 10–17% of eyes with pseudophakic retinal detachment have a history of vitreous loss during the cataract surgery. The pattern of retinal tears is similar to older studies of aphakia with less chance of large breaks, supratemporal breaks or presentation with VH and more inferonasal breaks than RRD in phakic eyes.[12] Surgical repair is by PPV.

Referral is as for RRD and depends on the presentation but will usually be as an emergency.

Table 5.2 Clinical features in atrophic hole RRD in young myopic patients

Sex	Females > males
Age	20–40 years
Refraction	Myopia
Bilateral	12% with bilateral RRD, retinal holes in the other eye (63%)
Fellow eye at presentation	10%
Onset	Slow
Vitreous	Attached
Retinal break type	Atrophic round
Retinal break size	Small
Retinal break position	Inferior > superior; temporal > nasal
Mean number of breaks	3.6
Multiple breaks: >1	70%
Fovea off	40%
PVR	Subretinal bands
Surgery	Explant

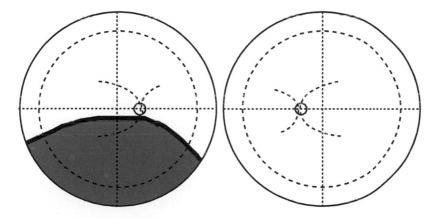

Figure 5.2 Round hole retinal detachments are usually inferior and slow to progress.

Table 5.3 shows a univariate comparison of various features of pseudophakic RRD with aged-related PVD-induced RRD; patients were older than 50 years.

APHAKIC RRD

Studies have been performed in this area in the 1960s and 1970s when intracapsular cataract surgery and aphakia were common.[13–17] Schepen's group in 1973 showed an increase in nasal breaks in aphakia versus phakia, 65% and 50.6%, respectively.[18] Similarly, Phillips,[19] in a group excluding vitreous loss, in 1963, found increased rates of breaks anteriorly, nasally and infero-nasally in aphakic retinal detachment compared with phakic retinal detachments.

Referral is as for RRD and depends on the presentation but will usually be as an emergency.

Table 5.3 Univariate comparison of various features of pseudophakic RRD with age-related PVD-induced RRD

Variable	Pseudophakic eyes	Phakic eyes	Significantly different
Age in years	69	64	Yes
Sex (female) (%)	31	41	Yes
Presenting visual acuity (mean)	20/180	20/160	
Duration of visual loss in days (mean)	15	31	
VH at presentation (%)	7	17	Yes
Presence of PVR (%)	14	14	
Number of breaks (mean)	2.5	2.7	
Fovea off (%)	64	55	
Small breaks (%)	56	46	Yes
Medium breaks (%)	60	59	
Large breaks (%)	13	27	Yes
Supratemporal break (%)	64	75	Yes
Inferotemporal break (%)	27	32	
Supranasal break (%)	38	38	
Inferonasal break (%)	21	14	Yes
Anterior break (%)	28	21	
Posterior break (%)	13	17	
Flat inferior break (%)	9	13	
Inferior breaks in the RRD	23	16	
Visual acuity at last follow-up (mean)	20/55	20/55	
Any RD at final follow-up (%)	5	4.0	
Oil in at final follow-up (%)	10	5	
Phthisis at final follow-up (%)	1	0	

RETINAL DIALYSIS

CLINICAL FEATURES

Retinal dialysis is a dehiscence of the anterior retina at the ora serrata. There is no PVD. The presence of a full vitreous means that the RRD progresses very slowly and often presents by coincidental observation or when the macula finally detaches. In the latter situation, because of the slow onset and delay in noticing the foveal detachment, visual recovery is seldom good. The chronicity results in subretinal fibrosis and retinal cysts but a lower rate of preretinal PVR.[20] If PVR is present, subretinal bands are more common than other types of PVR. The dialysis is usually stiff and smooth-edged, and the retinal detachment is often immobile (Figures 5.3 and 5.4).

A separation of the vitreous base from the retina is sometimes seen as a 'bucket handle' in the inner surface of the dialysis especially in traumatic cases. Blunt trauma has been associated with dialysis (Table 5.4)[21]. Occasionally, a retinal dialysis is seen a few days after a severe contusion injury, in which case, the dialysis and retina are mobile and progression is likely to be more rapid, therefore requiring more immediate referral. A history of trauma may be absent, and many presentations are spontaneous.[22] A familial basis has been sought but remains uncertain.[23,24]

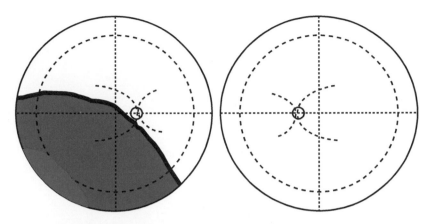

Figure 5.3 Inferotemporal retinal dialysis and detachment. The break is at the ora serrata and the vitreous is attached.

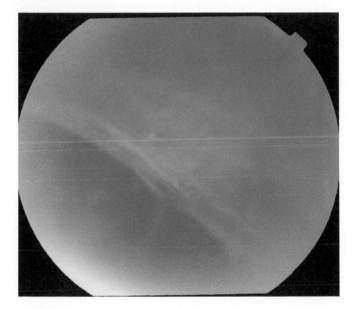

Figure 5.4 Retinal dialysis.

The most common sites for the dialysis are inferotemporal and superonasal. Fifty-six per cent of inferotemporal dialyses and 87% of superonasal dialyses have been associated with trauma.[25] Fourteen per cent of cases present bilaterally, in which case, the association with trauma is less. Atopic dermatitis[26] and Down's syndrome[27] have been associated with retinal dialysis.

The slow progression of retinal detachment means that most cases can be referred over a few days. If you are confident of signs of chronicity, e.g. pigment demarcation of the edge of the RRD, then even slower referral can be made. As with round hole retinal detachment, if the fovea has just detached, it is worth getting the patient seen soon to determine how quickly the fovea needs to be reattached to improve results (often, it takes a while for the patient to notice the central vision loss, however).

If the RRD appears immediately after trauma and the retina is mobile, an emergency referral is required.

Table 5.4 Clinical features in RRD from retinal dialysis

Sex	Males > females
Age	20–40 years
Refraction	Emmetropia
Fellow eye at presentation	8%
Onset	Slow
Vitreous	Attached
Retinal break type	Retinal dialysis
Retinal break size	Large and medium
Retinal break quadrant	Inferotemporal (superonasal more likely to be traumatic)
Median number of breaks	1
Multiple breaks: >1	30%
Fovea off	40%
PVR	Subretinal bands
Surgery	Explant

Source: *Can J Ophthalmol*, 49, Qiang Kwong T. et al., Characteristics of rhegmatogenous retinal detachments secondary to retinal dialyses, 196–9, Copyright (2014), with permission from Elsevier.

GIANT RETINAL DIALYSIS

This is a rare presentation in which the dialysis is more than 90°. The presentation in my experience has occurred in patients with an odd traumatic history such as patients who may injure their own eyes (e.g. schizophrenia) or patients who are under institutional care from neurological deficit (e.g. cerebral palsy).

PAR CILIARIS TEAR

This is a rare form of dialysis in which the tear is located in the pars plana. It occurs in severe blunt trauma and is usually seen in the superonasal quadrant. Consider the diagnosis in a child with a total shallow RRD of uncertain history (unfortunately usual in children), which is of unknown duration. These breaks are difficult to see and diagnose and, because of delay in presentation, often accompanied with PVR.

GIANT RETINAL TEAR

CLINICAL FEATURES

A giant retinal tear (GRT) is defined as a tear of more than 3 clock hours of the retina (or 90°) with PVD. They are rare with an incidence 0.091 per 100,000 in the United Kingdom.[28] The patients are often in the age of 20–50 years, more often male and present early, more frequently with the macula still on (55%)[28] compared to routine RRD. The vitreous is detached from the posterior pole and attached to the anterior portion of the retinal tear, thereby distinguishing from a dialysis. The tear can fold over on itself onto the retina. In addition, there may be radial slits at either end of the tear extending posteriorly. There may be satellite U-shaped breaks elsewhere in the retina (Figures 5.5 and 5.6).

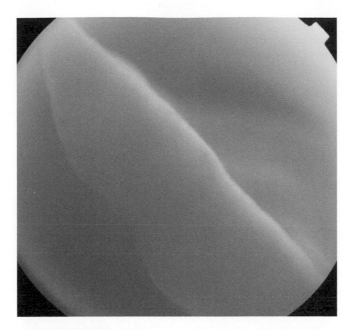

Figure 5.5 Very large retinal break is called a GRT and must be more than 90° of the retina.

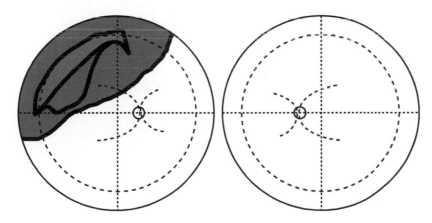

Figure 5.6 GRTs are larger than 90° (3 clock hours), often have slits at their ends and often fold on top of the retina.

A GRT may occur in isolation, usually in a myopic patient, but may also be present in hereditary vitreoretinal disorders such as Stickler's syndrome (14%)[29] or, rarely, in Marfan's syndrome.[30] In Stickler's syndrome, in particular, there is a risk of bilateral retinal tears in up to 40% of patients depending on the severity of the syndrome, and for this reason, some surgeons advocate prophylactic 360° cryotherapy to the fellow eye.[31]

A GRT can also occur as a result of trauma that is either penetrating or nonpenetrating.[32,33] Complicated anterior segment surgery may create GRT.[34,35]

Referral is as an emergency to prevent progression to macula off and reattach macula-off retinal detachments soon. In addition, these large tears are associated with PVR if left too long and should therefore be dealt with promptly.

STICKLER'S SYNDROME

This syndrome is characterised by the following:

- Myopia
- Paravascular lattice
- Dragging of the major vessels at the optic disc
- Veils or condensations of cortical vitreous around large lacunae (optically empty vitreous) or dehiscences in the gel
- Multiple posterior vitreoretinal adhesions

Stickler's syndrome has an autosomal dominant inheritance with highly variable penetrance, which means that patients are variably affected. A possible genetic abnormality has been identified at COL2A1.[36–38]

Systemic associations are as follows:

- High palate
- Characteristic facies with a flattened nasal bridge
- Short mandible and long philtre
- Arthralgia[39]

Retinal detachments are related to posterior paravascular vitreoretinal adhesions or to radially orientated post-equatorial lattice degeneration. Bilateral GRTs are common (Figure 5.7).

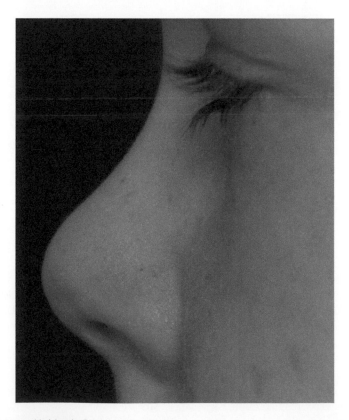

Figure 5.7 Flat nasal bridge in Stickler's syndrome.

OTHER EYE

Historically, the reported bilateral rate of GRTs is high, especially in Stickler's syndrome (25–40%). Some surgeons have advocated 360° cryotherapy retinopexy in the unaffected eye because of the risk of bilaterality,[40–42] reducing bilaterality to 6–10% in retrospective studies.[31,41]

RETINAL DETACHMENT IN HIGH MYOPES

CLINICAL FEATURES

Retinal breaks in the macula in emmetropia do not usually cause retinal detachment (e.g. senile macular holes). In highly myopic eyes, posterior breaks, especially at the macula or nasal to the optic disc, often associated with areas of chorioretinal atrophy and with posterior staphylomas cause retinal detachment. The detachment usually remains at the posterior pole, occasionally extending anteriorly. The ILM, vitreoschisis and partial vitreous separation[43] around the hole may be implicated in the pathogenesis of the retinal detachment because the surgical removal of the residual vitreous cortex and ILM during vitrectomy facilitates retinal reattachment. Once those tissues have been removed, the retina remains flat even if the hole is open post-operatively and untreated by retinopexy.[44] During a follow-up, 8.5% develop RRD in their fellow eyes in 5 years.[45]

In addition, the retina of the macula may become schitic with an associated drop in vision. If followed, these eyes can develop macular SRF or macular hole,[46] and the staphylomas progress.[47]

Macular retinoschisis without retinal break can be treated by vitrectomy[48–51] but with the risk of creating a foveal hole in some patients (Figures 5.8 and 5.9).

As an alternative to vitrectomy, a scleral buckle can be placed to produce a macular plombage to flatten the retina as an alternative to PPV.[52] Posterior pole buckles have also been used to slow the progression of myopia.[53] There is a tendency to shorten the eye with these buckles, but the distortion of vision may occur from the indent induced on the macula.

By definition, these present as a macula-off retinal detachment. Referral rates depend on the duration of loss of central vision. The quicker the retina is fixed in general, the better the visual recovery, but of course, those with macular hole have reduced prognosis. Other features such as myopic macular changes and chorioretinal atrophy also reduce the outcomes for vision (Figures 5.10 and 5.11).

RETINOSCHISIS-RELATED RETINAL DETACHMENT

CLINICAL FEATURES

The term *retinoschisis* refers to a process whereby fluid accumulates within the retinal neuro-epithelium to form a large intraretinal cyst, thereby splitting the retina. The cyst cavity has an inner leaf (in the vitreous cavity) and an outer leaf (on the RPE). Retinal breaks may develop in one or both of these leaves. When fluid passes through an inner leaf break and then an outer leaf breaks, the outer layer detaches from the pigment epithelium and the schisis is said to have progressed to a retinal detachment. Occasionally, fluid within the schisis can enter the subretinal space through the outer leaf break (without an inner leaf break) and very slowly lift the retina, giving a slow onset retinal detachment (Figure 5.12).

Retinoschises are classically divided into 'infantile' and senile varieties.

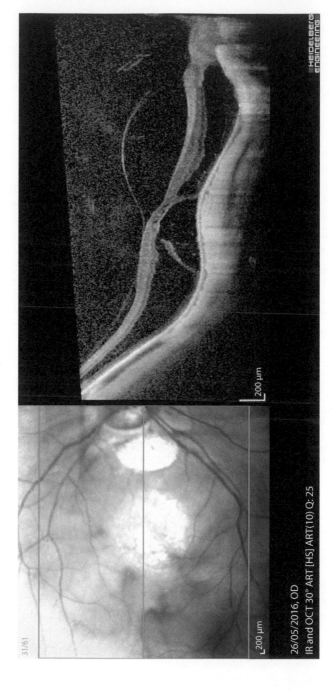

Figure 5.8 Macula of this myopic eye shows schisis and elevation.

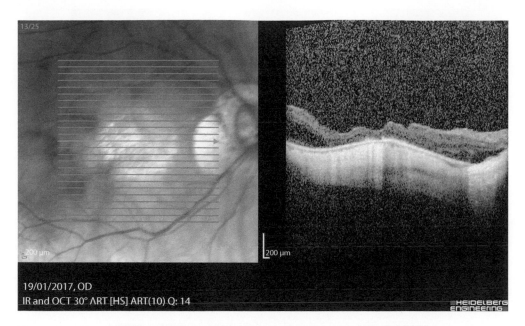

Figure 5.9 After surgery, the retina is flattened, but the retina is thin and vision is only slightly improved.

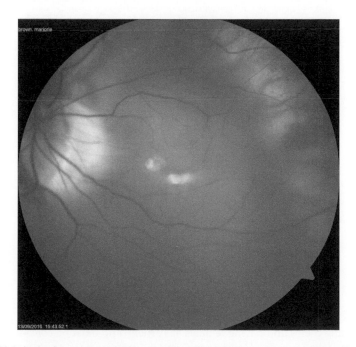

Figure 5.10 Hole in the fovea has created a macular retinal detachment in a patient with pathological high myopia.

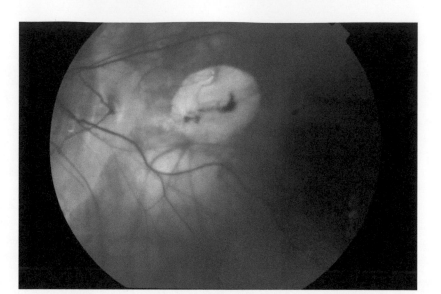

Figure 5.11 Retinal detachment at the posterior pole in a patient with pathological high myopia.

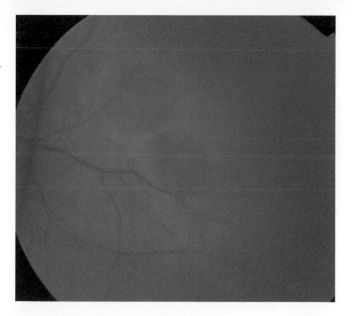

Figure 5.12 Outer leaf breaks in a patient with retinoschisis.

INFANTILE RETINOSCHISIS

Infantile retinoschisis is a rare disorder with an X-linked recessive mode of inheritance, therefore affecting young males and having females as carriers, and must be considered in the differential diagnosis when a young boy presents with retinal elevation. A common presentation is VH, while central vision may be impaired by associated foveal schisis. The inner leaf may be extremely thin because the split in the retina is at the level of the ganglion cells, with large breaks between the blood vessels. Progression to true RRD is unusual. The resolution of the macular schisis with restoration of the foveal dip has been described in a few patients after PPV.[54]

SENILE RETINOSCHISIS

Senile retinoschisis occurs after middle age, is usually bilateral, tends to be located inferotemporally and is frequently discovered during routine examination of the peripheral fundus. It is probably more common in hypermetropes. The split in the retina is in the outer plexiform layer, and therefore, the inner leaf is relatively thick. In most schisis, there are no retinal breaks and the outer leaf of the schisis often has a grey translucency with a mottled pattern. If present, outer leaf breaks tend to be large with rolled edges and may be pigmented, while inner leaf breaks are usually small and round. Most schisis will remain stable, and no intervention is required unless RRD occurs.[55–60]

DIFFERENTIATION OF RETINOSCHISIS FROM CHRONIC RRD

Differentiation from chronic retinal detachment (usually atrophic round hole RRD) may be difficult and primarily relies on experience and the ability of the observer to differentiate detached full-thickness retina from a thinner inner leaf. Other features help, however (see Table 5.5).

A pigmented demarcation line, often seen in chronic retinal detachment, may occasionally be seen in retinoschisis where haemorrhage into the cyst has occurred.

RETINAL DETACHMENT IN RETINOSCHISIS

Occasionally, a retinal detachment is seen advancing from the schisis; this advancing edge should consist of the full thickness of the retina and not an increase in the area of split retina, i.e. the schisis itself. The appearance of the retina should show a line where the thin inner leaf joins the thicker (and more opaque) full-thickness retina. OCT can be used to differentiate the schitic retina from the full-thickness elevated retina if the elevation is extending posteriorly (Figures 5.13 and 5.14).

Two types are described:

- Slow type from egress of the fluid in the cyst cavity through the outer leaf breaks and into the subretinal space: There are no inner leaf breaks. These can be referred in a week or two if you are confident of the diagnosis.
- Fast type, with rapid onset RRD in schisis, which has inner and outer leaves, breaks: Vitreous cavity fluid can enter the subretinal space producing a more rapid accumulation of SRF. These will require rapid referral as with any acute RRD.

Table 5.5 Comparisons between chronic RRD and retinoschisis

Retinoschisis	Chronic retinal detachment
Retina moves inwards on indentation	Retina does not move inwards
Outer leaf breaks and retina on outer surface visible	Bare RPE on outer wall
Absolute visual field defect; patient cannot see indenter when placed in front of indirect ophthalmoscope illumination	Relative visual field defect; patient can see T bar of indenter
Patient unaware of visual field loss	Patient aware of area of field loss
Often hyperopic	Often myopic
No pigment in vitreous	Pigment in the vitreous
Usually no pigmented demarcation line (unless there has previously been a bleed into the cyst)	Demarcation line sometimes present

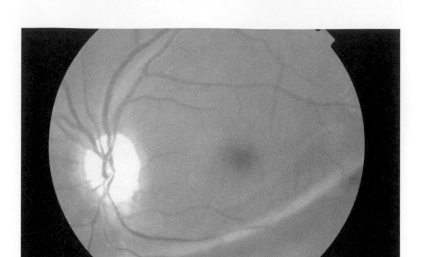

Figure 5.13 Retinal detachment in a patient with X-linked retinoschisis.

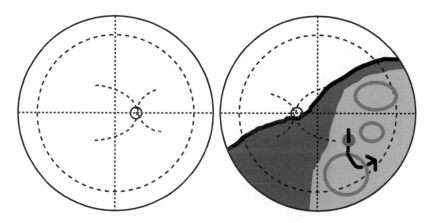

Figure 5.14 Retinal detachment (*blue*) secondary to retinoschisis (*light blue*) occurs when fluid passes through a small hole (*solid red*) in the inner leaf of the schisis and then through larger holes (*red outlines*) in the outer leaf of the schisis.

JUVENILE RETINAL DETACHMENT

Children occasionally present with RRD, usually with a predisposing factor such as trauma, high myopia, Stickler's syndrome, previous intraocular surgery, familial exudative vitreoretinopathy, uveitis and previous retinopathy of prematurity.[61,62] The frequency of bilateral vision-threatening abnormalities in these patients is reportedly high at 89%.[63] PVR rates are also high (40%) because of the slow recognition of the loss of the vision and, therefore, late presentation. Both final retinal reattachment rates and visual acuity outcomes are lower than those for adult surgery.

Be wary of a child with severe reduction of vision and no history of the loss of vision; examination of the retina may reveal a retinal detachment.

ATOPIC DERMATITIS

This has been associated with RRD in 2.2% of patients in Japan[64] with a high incidence of cataract and PVR.

REFRACTIVE SURGERY

Although RRD has been described to be associated with Lasik,[65] the causal relationship remains uncertain. In one study, only 17 patients had RRD from 1 to 36 months after Lasik out of 31,739 patients, which is likely equivalent to a normal population of myopic patients.[66]

CONGENITAL CATARACT

Patients with prior history for congenital cataract may present with RRD especially if they have had surgery for the cataract. The presentation is usually similar to other acute retinal detachments and can be referred in a similar manner (Figure 5.15).

OTHERS

RRD can complicate many other conditions, which are more fully described elsewhere in this book. Any condition which causes PVD in the presence of vitreoretinal adhesions or which injures the retina by causing a full-thickness break can potentially cause RRD, such as the following:

- Uveitis
- Trauma
- Viral retinitis
- Retinal vein occlusion

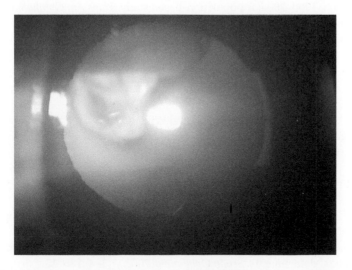

Figure 5.15 Sommerung's ring in an eye with previous congenital cataract extractions.

- von Hippel–Lindau disease
- Sickle cell disease
- Dropped nucleus
- Needle-stick injury
- Vitreoretinal surgery
- Retinopathy of prematurity

REFERENCES

1. Ung, T., Comer, M. B., Ang, A. J. et al. Clinical features and surgical management of retinal detachment secondary to round retinal holes. *Eye (Lond)* 2005;19(6):665–9.
2. Gonzales, C. R., Gupta, A., Schwartz, S. D. and Kreiger, A. E. The fellow eye of patients with rhegmatogenous retinal detachment. *Ophthalmology* 2004;111(3):518–21.
3. Gonzales, C. R., Gupta, A., Schwartz, S. D. and Kreiger, A. E. The fellow eye of patients with phakic rhegmatogenous retinal detachment from atrophic holes of lattice degeneration without posterior vitreous detachment. *Br J Ophthalmol* 2004;88(11):1400–2.
4. Javitt, J. C., Vitale, S., Canner, J. K. et al. National outcomes of cataract extraction. I. Retinal detachment after inpatient surgery. *Ophthalmology* 1991;98(6):895–902.
5. Javitt, J. C., Tielsch, J. M., Canner, J. K. et al. National outcomes of cataract extraction: Increased risk of retinal complications associated with Nd:YAG laser capsulotomy: The Cataract Patient Outcomes Research Team. *Ophthalmology* 1992;99(10):1487–97.
6. Sheu, S. J., Ger, L. P. and Ho, W. L. Late increased risk of retinal detachment after cataract extraction. *Am J Ophthalmol* 2010;149(1):113–9.
7. Boberg-Ans, G., Villumsen, J. and Henning, V. Retinal detachment after phacoemulsification cataract extraction. *J Cataract Refract Surg* 2003;29(7):1333–8.
8. Boberg-Ans, G., Henning, V., Villumsen, J. and la Cour, M. Long-term incidence of rhegmatogenous retinal detachment and survival in a defined population undergoing standardized phacoemulsification surgery. *Acta Ophthalmol Scand* 2006;84(5):613–8.
9. Erie, J. C., Raecker, M. E., Baratz, K. H. et al. Risk of retinal detachment after cataract extraction, 1980–2004: A population-based study. *Trans Am Ophthalmol Soc* 2006;104:167–75.
10. Lois, N. and Wong, D. Pseudophakic retinal detachment. *Surv Ophthalmol* 2003;48(5):467–87.
11. Bradford, J. D., Wilkinson, C. P. and Fransen, S. R. Pseudophakic retinal detachments: The relationships between retinal tears and the time following cataract surgery at which they occur. *Retina* 1989;9(3):181–6.
12. Mahroo, O. A., Dybowski, R., Wong, R. and Williamson, T. H. Characteristics of rhegmatogenous retinal detachment in pseudophakic and phakic eyes. *Eye (Lond)* 2012;26(8):1114–21.
13. Menezo, J. L., Frances, J. and Reynolds, R. S. Number and shape of tears in aphakic retinal detachment: Its relationship with different surgical techniques of cataract extraction. *Mod Probl Ophthalmol* 1977;18:457–63.
14. Snyder, W. B., Bernstein, I., Fuller, D. et al. Retinal detachment and pseudophakia. *Ophthalmology* 1979;86(2):229–41.
15. Ramos, M., Kruger, E. F. and Lashkari, K. Biostatistical analysis of pseudophakic and aphakic retinal detachments. *Semin Ophthalmol* 2002;17(3–4):206–13.

16. McDonnell, P. J., Patel, A. and Green, W. R. Comparison of intracapsular and extra-capsular cataract surgery: Histopathologic study of eyes obtained postmortem. *Ophthalmology* 1985;92(9):1208–25.

17. Tuft, S. J., Minassian, D. and Sullivan, P. Risk factors for retinal detachment after cataract surgery: A case-control study. *Ophthalmology* 2006;113(4):650–6.

18. Yoshida, A., Ogasawara, H., Jalkh, A. E. et al. Retinal detachment after cataract surgery: Surgical results. *Ophthalmology* 1992;99(3):460–5.

19. Phillips, C. I. Distribution of breaks in aphakic and 'senile' eyes with retinal detachments. *Br J Ophthalmol* 1963;47:744–52.

20. Kennedy, C. J., Parker, C. E. and McAllister, I. L. Retinal detachment caused by retinal dialysis. *Aust NZ J Ophthalmol* 1997;25(1):25–30.

21. Qiang Kwong, T., Shunmugam, M. and Williamson, T. H. Characteristics of rhegmatogenous retinal detachments secondary to retinal dialyses. *Can J Ophthalmol* 2014;49(2):196–9.

22. Kinyoun, J. L. and Knobloch, W. H. Idiopathic retinal dialysis. *Retina* 1984;4(1):9–14.

23. Verdaguer, T. J., Rojas, B. and Lechuga, M. Genetical studies in nontraumatic retinal dialysis. *Mod Probl Ophthalmol* 1975;15:34–9.

24. Ross, W. H. Retinal dialysis: Lack of evidence for a genetic cause. *Can J Ophthalmol* 1991;26(6):309–12.

25. Zion, V. M. and Burton, T. C. Retinal dialysis. *Arch Ophthalmol* 1980;98(11):1971–4.

26. Katsura, H. and Hida, T. Atopic dermatitis: Retinal detachment associated with atopic dermatitis. *Retina* 1984;4(3):148–51.

27. Ahmad, A. and Pruett, R. C. The fundus in mongolism. *Arch Ophthalmol* 1976;94(5):772–6.

28. Ang, G. S., Townend, J. and Lois, N. Epidemiology of giant retinal tears in the United Kingdom: The British Giant Retinal Tear Epidemiology Eye Study (BGEES). *Invest Ophthalmol Vis Sci* 2010;51(9):4781–7.

29. Billington, B. M., Leaver, P. K. and McLeod, D. Management of retinal detachment in the Wagner-Stickler syndrome. *Trans Ophthalmol Soc UK* 1985;104 (Pt 8):875–9.

30. Sharma, T., Gopal, L., Shanmugam, M. P. et al. Retinal detachment in Marfan syndrome: Clinical characteristics and surgical outcome. *Retina* 2002;22(4):423–8.

31. Wolfensberger, T. J., Aylward, G. W. and Leaver, P. K. Prophylactic 360 degrees cryotherapy in fellow eyes of patients with spontaneous giant retinal tears. *Ophthalmology* 2003;110(6):1175–7.

32. Duguid, I. G. and Leaver, P. K. Giant retinal tears resulting from eye gouging in rugby football. *Br J Sports Med* 2000;34(1):65–6.

33. Aylward, G. W., Cooling, R. J. and Leaver, P. K. Trauma-induced retinal detachment associated with giant retinal tears. *Retina* 1993;13(2):136–41.

34. McLeod, D. Giant retinal tears after central vitrectomy. *Br J Ophthalmol* 1985;69(2):96–8.

35. Aaberg, T. M. Jr., Rubsamen, P. E., Flynn, H. W. Jr. et al. Giant retinal tear as a complication of attempted removal of intravitreal lens fragments during cataract surgery. *Am J Ophthalmol* 1997;124(2):222–6.

36. Richards, A. J., Meredith, S., Poulson, A. et al. A novel mutation of COL2A1 resulting in dominantly inherited rhegmatogenous retinal detachment. *Invest Ophthalmol Vis Sci* 2005;46(2):663–8.

37. Richards, A. J., Martin, S., Yates, J. R. et al. COL2A1 exon 2 mutations: Relevance to the Stickler and Wagner syndromes. *Br J Ophthalmol* 2000;84(4):364–71.

38. Snead, M. P. and Yates, J. R. Clinical and molecular genetics of Stickler syndrome. *J Med Genet* 1999;36(5):353–9.

39. Spallone, A. Stickler's syndrome: A study of 12 families. *Br J Ophthalmol* 1987;71(7):504–9.
40. Ambresin, A., Wolfensberger, T. J. and Bovey, E. H. Management of giant retinal tears with vitrectomy, internal tamponade, and peripheral 360 degrees retinal photocoagulation. *Retina* 2003;23(5):622–8.
41. Ang, A., Poulson, A. V., Goodburn, S. F. et al. Retinal detachment and prophylaxis in type 1 Stickler syndrome. *Ophthalmology* 2008;115(1):164–8.
42. Ang, G. S., Townend, J. and Lois, N. Interventions for prevention of giant retinal tear in the fellow eye. *Cochrane Database Syst Rev* 2009(2):CD006909.
43. Matsumura, N., Ikuno, Y. and Tano, Y. Posterior vitreous detachment and macular hole formation in myopic foveoschisis. *Am J Ophthalmol* 2004;138(6):1071–3.
44. Ikuno, Y., Sayanagi, K., Oshima T. et al. Optical coherence tomographic findings of macular holes and retinal detachment after vitrectomy in highly myopic eyes. *Am J Ophthalmol* 2003;136(3):477–81.
45. Oie, Y. and Emi, K. Incidence of fellow eye retinal detachment resulting from macular hole. *Am J Ophthalmol* 2007;143(2):203–5.
46. Shimada, N., Ohno-Matsui, K., Baba, T. et al. Natural course of macular retinoschisis in highly myopic eyes without macular hole or retinal detachment. *Am J Ophthalmol* 2006;142(3):497–500.
47. Hsiang, H. W., Ohno-Matsui, K., Shimada, N. et al. Clinical characteristics of posterior staphyloma in eyes with pathologic myopia. *Am J Ophthalmol* 2008;146(1):102–10.
48. Kuhn, F. Internal limiting membrane removal for macular detachment in highly myopic eyes. *Am J Ophthalmol* 2003;135(4):547–9.
49. Ikuno, Y., Sayanagi, K., Ohji, M. et al. Vitrectomy and internal limiting membrane peeling for myopic foveoschisis. *Am J Ophthalmol* 2004;137(4):719–24.
50. Kobayashi, H. and Kishi, S. Vitreous surgery for highly myopic eyes with foveal detachment and retinoschisis. *Ophthalmology* 2003;110(9):1702–7.
51. Kanda, S., Uemura, A., Sakamoto, Y. and Kita, H. Vitrectomy with internal limiting membrane peeling for macular retinoschisis and retinal detachment without macular hole in highly myopic eyes. *Am J Ophthalmol* 2003;136(1):177–80.
52. Baba, T., Tanaka, S., Maesawa, A. et al. Scleral buckling with macular plombe for eyes with myopic macular retinoschisis and retinal detachment without macular hole. *Am J Ophthalmol* 2006;142(3):483–7.
53. Ward, B., Tarutta, E. P. and Mayer, M. J. The efficacy and safety of posterior pole buckles in the control of progressive high myopia. *Eye (Lond)* 2009;23(12):2169–74.
54. Ikeda, F., Iida, T. and Kishi, S. Resolution of retinoschisis after vitreous surgery in X-linked retinoschisis. *Ophthalmology* 2008;115(4):718–22 e1.
55. Byer, N. E. Clinical study of senile retinoschisis. *Arch Ophthalmol* 1968;79(1):36–44.
56. Byer, N. E. Long-term natural history study of senile retinoschisis with implications for management. *Ophthalmology* 1986;93(9):1127–37.
57. Byer, N. E. The natural history of senile retinoschisis. *Trans Am Acad Ophthalmol Otolaryngol* 1976;81(3 Pt 1):458–71.
58. Byer, N. E. The natural history of senile retinoschisis. *Mod Probl Ophthalmol* 1977;18:304–11.
59. Byer, N. E. Perspectives on the management of the complications of senile retinoschisis. *Eye* 2002;16(4):359–64.
60. Byer, N. E. Spontaneous regression of senile retinoschisis. *Arch Ophthalmol* 1972;88(2):207–9.

61. Weinberg, D. V., Lyon, A. T., Greenwald, M. J. and Mets, M. B. Rhegmatogenous retinal detachments in children: Risk factors and surgical outcomes. *Ophthalmology* 2003;110(9):1708–13.

62. Akabane, N., Yamamoto, S., Tsukahara, I. et al. Surgical outcomes in juvenile retinal detachment. *Jpn J Ophthalmol* 2001;45(4):409–11.

63. Fivgas, G. D. and Capone, A. Jr. Pediatric rhegmatogenous retinal detachment. *Retina* 2001;21(2):101–6.

64. Hida, T., Tano, Y., Okinami, S. et al. Multicenter retrospective study of retinal detachment associated with atopic dermatitis. *Jpn J Ophthalmol* 2000;44(4):407–18.

65. Farah, M. E., Hofling-Lima, A. L. and Nascimento, E. Early rhegmatogenous retinal detachment following laser in situ keratomileusis for high myopia. *J Refract Surg* 2000;16(6):739–43.

66. Arevalo, J. F., Ramirez, E., Suarez, E. et al. Rhegmatogenous retinal detachment in myopic eyes after laser in situ keratomileusis: Frequency, characteristics, and mechanism. *J Cataract Refract Surg* 2001;27(5):674–80.

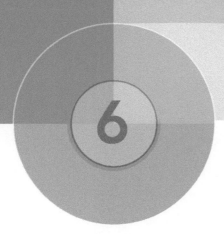

Macular disorders

6

INTRODUCTION

The macula is a common site of symptomatic retinal pathology requiring vitreoretinal intervention. PVD is implicated in the production of the most common vitreoretinal macular disorders.

IDIOPATHIC MACULAR HOLE

CLINICAL FEATURES

INTRODUCTION

Age-related macular hole is a tangential dehiscence of the neuroretinal layer of the retina at the fovea:

- Occurs in middle-aged or elderly patients
- Occurs in 3.3 females:1 male
- Occurs 7.8/100,000 population[1]
- Bilateral in 12–13% in 2 years after presentation in one eye[2]

Patients' symptoms consist of blurred vision or distortion. In the early stages (grade 1), the patient sees a small central grey patch in their central vision, and because the receptors are not yet displaced, distortion of the image is usually absent. Distortion becomes a feature as the fovea splits apart and the photoreceptors are moved outwards onto the rim of the hole (grades 2 and 3). Typically, the features at the centre of the patient's visual image (e.g. the nose of a face) are reduced in size (micropsia). The brain receives fewer signals than it should in the centre of the macula because the receptors are spread apart on the rim of the macular hole. The patient's visual system interprets this as a falsely small image centrally, hence the reduction in the size of the nose when the patient looks at a face. Eventually, over time the receptors at the edge of the hole will stop functioning (grades 3 and 4), and the patient will have a central scotoma and the nose will be missing (Figure 6.1).

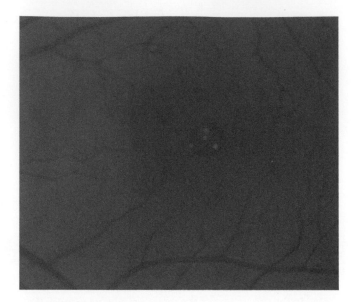

Figure 6.1 Colour image of a macular hole.

WATZKE–ALLEN TEST

The phenomena of distortion and loss of vision are exploited in the Watzke-Allen test.[3] To perform this test, shine a thin line of light vertically via the slit lamp biomicroscope across the macular hole.

Ask the patient to describe the line of light.

There are three possibilities:

- Straight: an intact fovea
- Narrowing centrally: separated but functioning foveal receptors
- Gap centrally[3]: loss of function of the receptors[4]

It is the process of vitreous detachment that creates the macular hole. The separation of the vitreous is often visible on OCT of the macula. A prefoveal operculum may be visible in the early stages and is not thought to be primarily retinal tissue.[5,6]

GRADING

The Gass grading system is still used to describe macular holes because it provides a guide to surgical success and visual outcome. The grading system devised by Gass relates to ophthalmoscopy and not to OCT findings.

- Grade 1: The hole commences as a foveal intraretinal cyst[7] (1A) or a ring of cysts (1B), seen as a central yellow spot or ring of spots,[8–10] at which point, the patient may be asymptomatic or have mild blur or distortion (Figures 6.2 through 6.9).
- Grade 2: A small crescentic or round hole less than 400 μm.
- Grade 3: A large round hole of more than 400 μm diameter (Figures 6.10 and 6.11).
- Grade 4: A hole with an associated PVD (Figure 6.12).

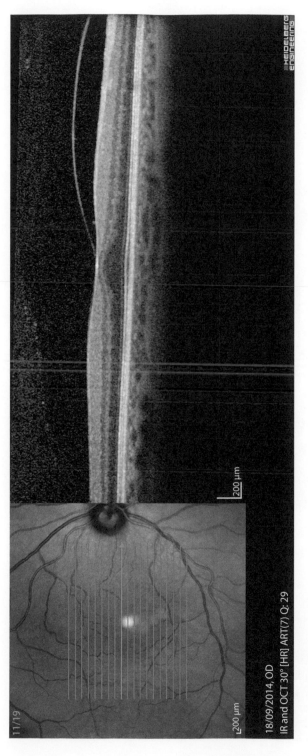

18/09/2014, OD

IR and OCT 30° [HR] ART(7) Q: 29

Figure 6.2 Early vitreoretinal separation.

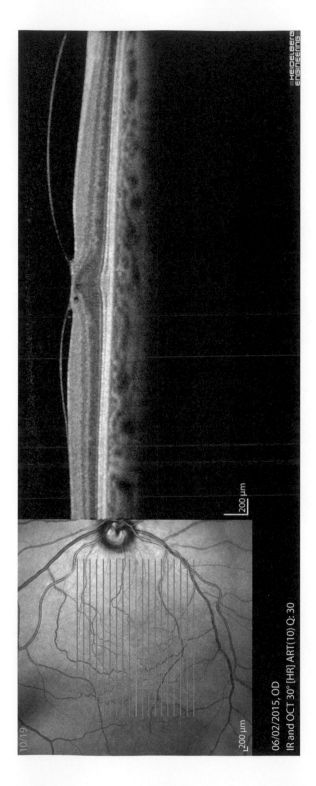

06/02/2015, OD

IR and OCT 30° [HR] ART(10) Q: 30

Figure 6.3 Separation progresses and produces some traction on the fovea.

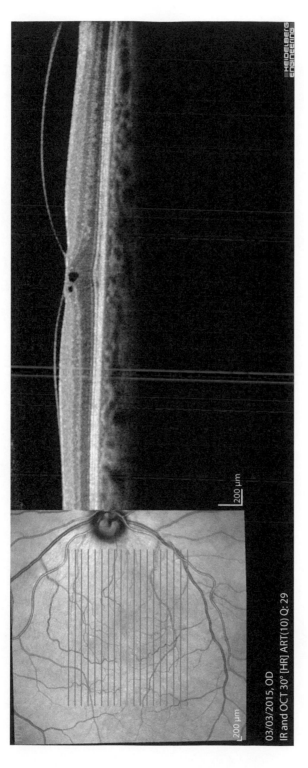

03/03/2015, OD
IR and OCT 30° [HR] ART(10) Q: 29

Figure 6.4 Eventually, a grade 1 macular hole has appeared.

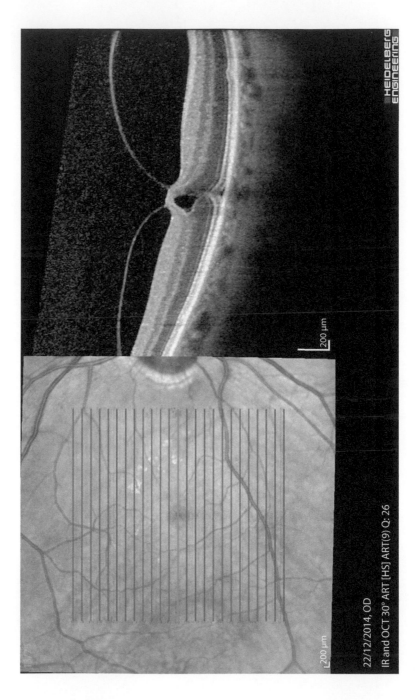

22/12/2014, OD

IR and OCT 30° ART [HS] ART(9) Q: 26

200 µm

200 µm

HEIDELBERG
ENGINEERING

Figure 6.5 Grade 1 macular hole, which spontaneously improves after separation of the vitreous.

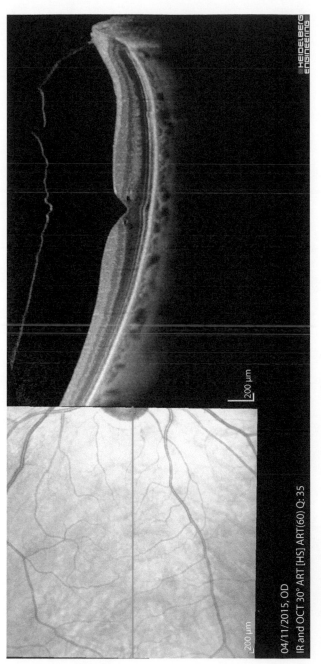

04/11/2015, OD
IR and OCT 30° ART [HS] ART(60) Q: 35

Figure 6.6 After separation of the vitreous from the fovea, the retina recovers to a better configuration.

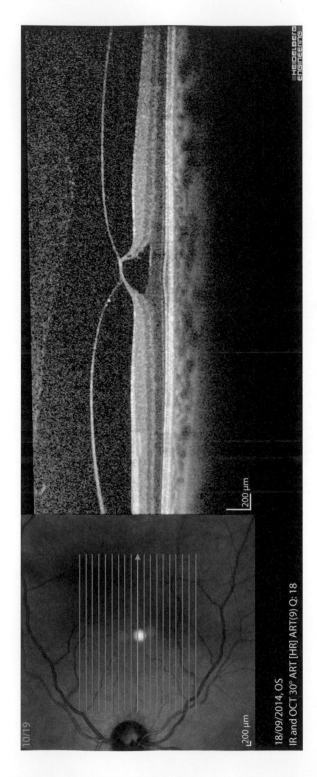

Figure 6.7 Grade 1 macular hole with the vitreous attached to the inner retina and a cyst in the fovea.

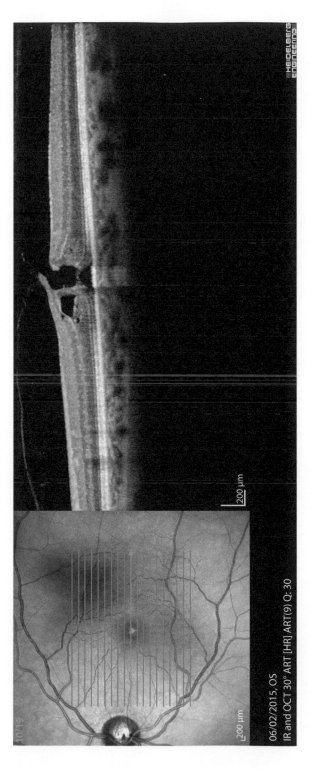

06/02/2015, OS
IR and OCT 30° ART [HR] ART(9) Q: 30

Figure 6.8 Cyst is converting into a full-thickness macular hole.

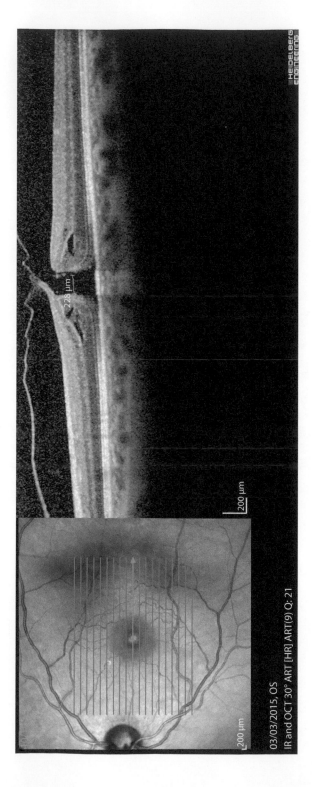

Figure 6.9 Hole has progressed into a full-thickness hole of grade 2 size (<400 μm).

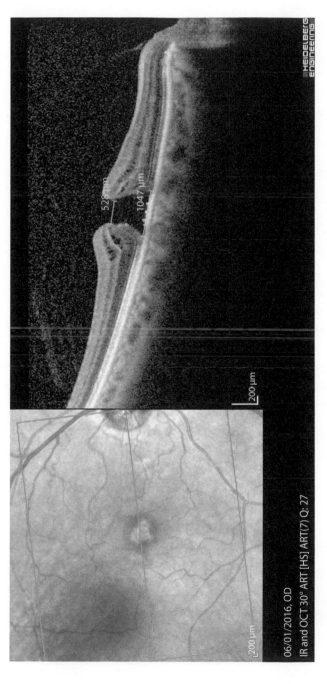

Figure 6.10 Grade 3 macular hole. The vitreous is attached to the optic nerve head and the hole is larger than 400 μm.

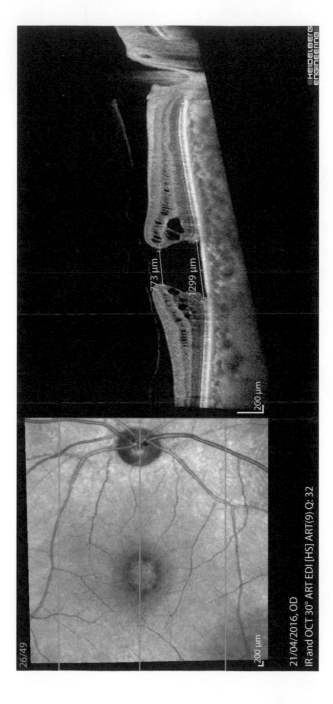

Figure 6.11 Large grade 3 macular hole. The size will reduce the chance of success of the surgery.

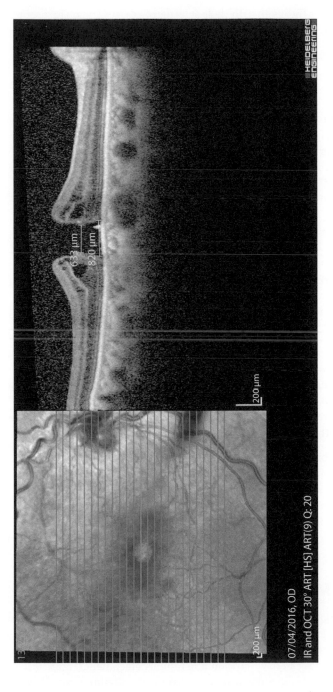

Figure 6.12 Grade 4 macular hole with separation of the vitreous from the optic disc. The hole is large, which, in combination with long duration, may indicate a poor visual prognosis and higher surgical failure rate.

113

A microseparation of the vitreous in an eye with a full-thickness hole would be graded as grade 3, not a grade 4, if no PVD is seen on ophthalmoscopy, e.g. evidenced by a Weiss ring.

Use OCT to measure the width of the hole at its narrowest separation to discriminate grades 2 and 3. Also, measure the base of the hole at the RPE. A larger base is associated with a poorer visual outcome.[11]

NATURAL HISTORY

- Grade 1 holes progress to full-thickness holes in 40% of cases,[12] with holes with poorer vision more likely to progress.[13]
- Seventy-four per cent of grade 2 holes progress to grade 3 or 4 in 6–12 months.[14]
- Spontaneous closure can occur, in 11.5% of grade 2 holes[15] and 4% of grade 3 and 4 holes.[16]
- At 5 years, there is a 75% chance of 20/200 vision or worse.[2,17]

OPTICAL COHERENCE TOMOGRAPHY

OCT is essential for confirming the diagnosis and to examine the other eye.[18,19] OCT images discriminate partial thickness lamellar 'holes' and pseudoholes (from ERM) from full-thickness macular holes.

OCT features the following:

- In a grade 1 hole, the posterior hyaloid pulls on the fovea causing an intraretinal cyst.
- In a grade 2 hole, the retina splits open and a small full thickness hole appears, often with the vitreous still attached to one edge.[20]
- In a grade 3 hole, the vitreous may be separated (but visible on the OCT) and the hole increased in size.
- The occult separation of the vitreous detectable on OCT is seen in 74% of grade 2 and 3 holes and is attached to the disc margin in 33%.[20,21]

The visible membrane on the posterior hyaloid probably consists of vitreous cortex with fragments of ILM.[22] The fellow eye shows the separation of the vitreous on OCT in 31%, indicating that the eye is safe from development of macular hole in the future.

Grade 0 macular holes are seen as a vitreous separation on OCT but with persistent attachment of the vitreous to the fovea (Figure 6.13). It is present in 29% of the contralateral eyes of patients with macular holes. In one study, 46% of eyes with Grade 0 progressed to macular hole at 2 years compared with 6% in those with no vitreous attachments (Figure 6.14).[23]

SECONDARY MACULAR HOLES

Severe contusion injury from blunt trauma to the eye can result in secondary macular holes.[24] These are reported to have a high spontaneous closure rate (50%) in the first few months; therefore, it is possible to wait a few months from the trauma before surgical intervention.[25] Traumatic macular holes can have surrounding retinal detachment (Figure 6.15).[26]

RRD may create a secondary macular hole. Yttrium aluminium garnet laser injury has been associated with hole formation.[27] Retinal pathologies such as sickle cell retinopathy and von Hippel–Lindau disease can produce macular holes.

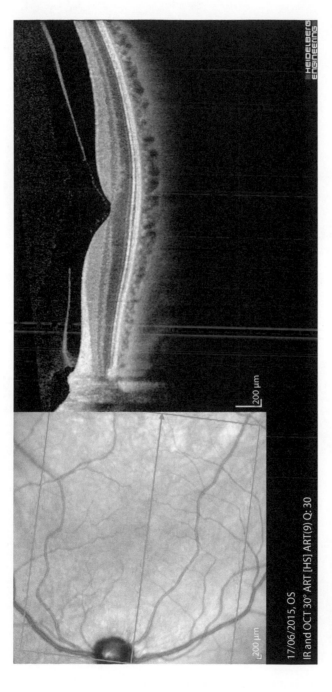

Figure 6.13 Grade 0 macular hole in the fellow eye of a patient with full-thickness macular hole in the other eye. This eye is at much higher risk of developing macular hole than an eye in which the vitreous has already separated.

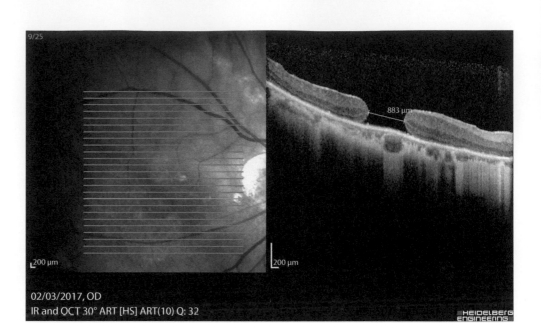

9/25

883 µm

200 µm

200 µm

02/03/2017, OD
IR and OCT 30° ART [HS] ART(10) Q: 32

HEIDELBERG
ENGINEERING

Figure 6.14 Large chronic macular hole with flat edges, which will not do well after surgery with a low closure rate.

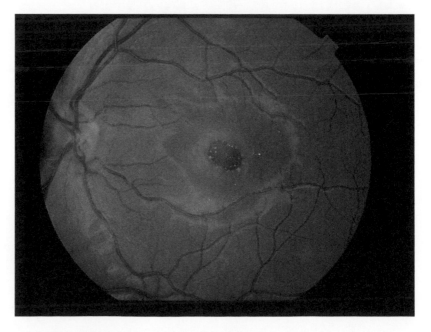

Figure 6.15 Large macular hole from blunt trauma to the eye.

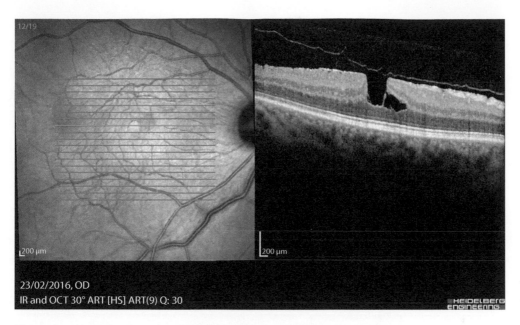

Figure 6.16 Lamellar dissection of the fovea with some ERM.

LAMELLAR AND PARTIAL THICKNESS HOLES

On some occasions, only the inner retina separates and the outer retina remains intact, producing a partial thickness hole with mild reduction of vision. They are most often associated with ERM. Lamellar holes should be discriminated from pseudoholes, which are holes in an ERM over the fovea with the underlying retina not affected.[28–34] PPV has been combined with ERM peel and ILM peel in patients with lamellar holes. When lamellar holes are left alone, the patient often experiences further slow deterioration of vision over the years to 20/120. Lamellar holes have also been described after chronic cystoid macular oedema (CMO) in diabetes or after cataract surgery and are associated with idiopathic retinal telangiectasia (Figure 6.16).[2,30–32]

Referral for surgery can be considered, but surgical outcomes are not well established.[34]

PARS PLANA VITRECTOMY

Surgery is successful in closing the hole. A very thin natural membrane called the ILM is often removed at surgery. A gas bubble is used to apply surface tension forces onto the hole to encourage it to close. The gas bubble can last for 3–9 weeks depending on its constituents. This reduces the patient's vision until the bubble has self-absorbed. Patients are advised not to fly (or go to higher altitude) with a gas bubble in situ, and if a general anaesthetic is required, the anaesthetist must be made aware of the gas bubble to avoid certain gas usage such as nitrous dioxide. Both of these scenarios can cause catastrophic rises in IOP (Figures 6.17 through 6.20).

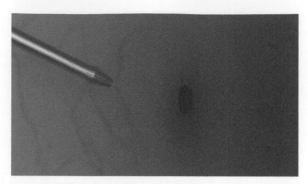

Figure 6.17 Removal of the ILM.

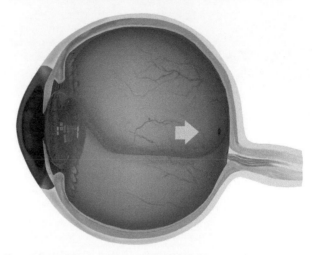

Figure 6.18 Inserting a gas bubble into the eye helps close the macular hole probably due to surface tension of the bubble on the retina.

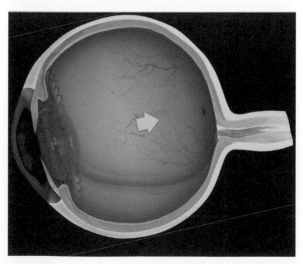

Figure 6.19 Gas bubble can be made to contact the macular hole with the eye looking slightly downwards.

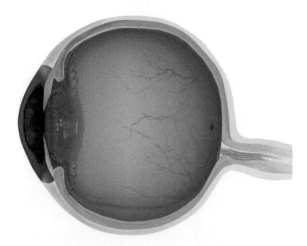

Figure 6.20 Larger gas bubble will contact the macula in the upright position.

MICROPLASMIN

Enzymatic vitreolysis showed promise as a method of inducing vitreal separation and may have a role for treating grade 0–2 macular holes. Microplasmin (125 µg) is injected intravitreally to induce separation in up to 44% of patients with vitreomacular adhesion.[35] Real-world results do not seem to have matched the results of the microplasmin for intravitreal injection (MIVI) trials with increased complication rates such as retinal detachment, outer retinal toxicity and loss of vision. Therefore, the impact of the therapy on the management of vitreomacular traction has been less than initially expected (Figures 6.21 and 6.22).[36]

REFERRAL

As with most retinal conditions, the success rate of interventions in macular hole is time dependent. Small early holes will close more often and with better visual results than large old ones.[37]

Unsurprisingly, the mean duration of symptoms relates to the grade of hole ($N = 351$):

- Grade 2: 0.53 years (standard deviation [SD] 0.43)
- Grade 3: 0.79 years (SD 0.68)
- Grade 4P: 1.20 years (SD 1.26)

Early holes achieve better final vision, e.g. better than 0.3 logMar (20/40):

- Grade 2: 37.4%
- Grade 3: 11.6%
- Grade 4: 15.4%

Therefore, the sooner the patient is seen and operated upon, the better. Macular holes tend to develop over months, and often, the patient takes some time to notice that the vision in one eye has reduced. The referral can be made by routine referral pattern as long as the local system is efficient enough to see the patient within 1–2 months. Where the hole is large and old, e.g. over 1 year, then the poorer surgical results for visual recovery can be discussed. Note that if the hole can be closed, a visual improvement may be seen even with grade 4 holes; therefore, the patient may wish to try to obtain visual improvement through surgery despite the low closure rate. Other methods such as reverse ILM flap surgery can be offered for old large eyes (Figures 6.23 through 6.25) (Table 6.1).[38]

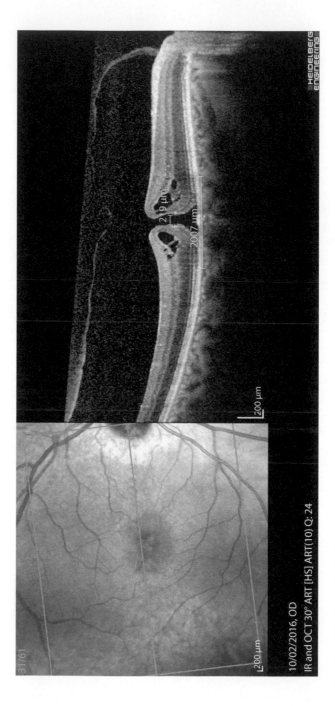

Figure 6.21 Macular hole not closed after plasmin injection, which shows some weakening of the receptors in the foveal area.

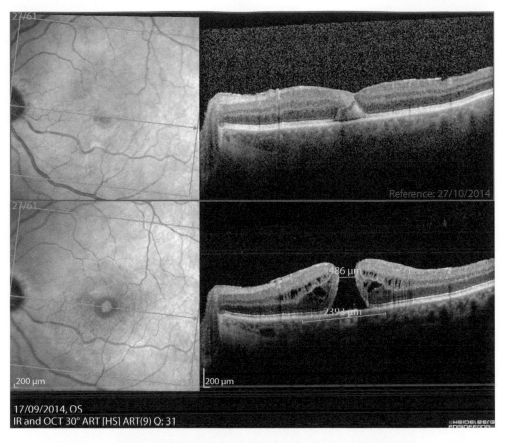

Figure 6.22 Macular hole in which plasmin has failed to close the hole (bottom) is treated by surgery, but the retina is not as healthy as might be expected despite closure of the hole (top).

MACULAR PUCKER AND VITREOMACULAR TRACTION

CLINICAL FEATURES

Idiopathic ERM includes the following conditions:

- Macular pucker: ERM with wrinkling of the retina or ERM
- Cellophane maculopathy: Thin sheet of ERM without significant retinal distortion

ERM is stimulated by PVD. The PVD may damage the ILM, stimulating fibrosis.[39,40] The membrane produces contracts and distorts the retina,[41,42] reducing the vision. ERMs in the macula have been described in 29% of people over the age of 45 years and increased in the Chinese population.[43,44]

The patient notices a blur of the vision, distortion and macropsia (increased image size) as the membrane contracts the retina centrally. The membrane is seen on biomicroscopy as a reflective sheet (cellophane) or as a thick opaque membrane. The retinal arcades may be tortuous. A pseudohole in the central membrane should be discriminated from a full-thickness hole in the retina (macular hole) by a negative Watzke–Allen test[45,46] and by performing an OCT

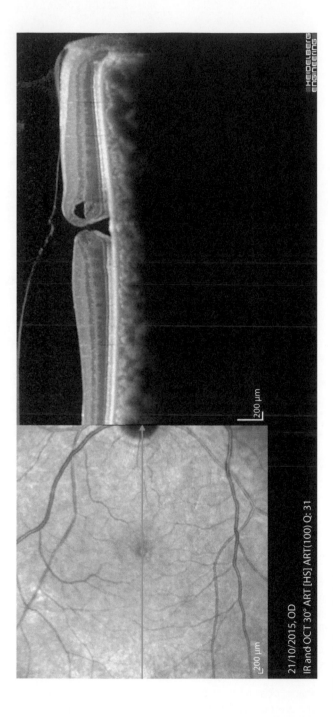

21/10/2015, OD

IR and OCT 30° ART [HS] ART(100) Q: 31

Figure 6.23 Grade 2 macular hole.

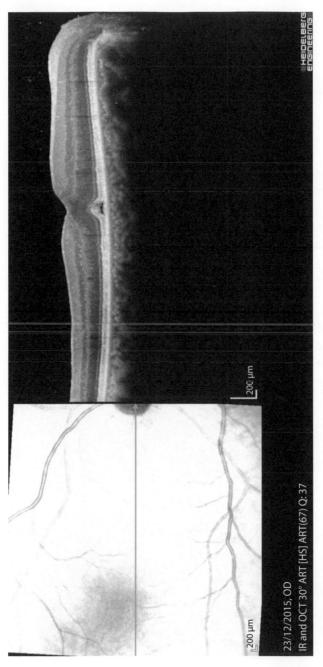

200 µm

200 µm

23/12/2015, OD
IR and OCT 30° ART [HS] ART(67) Q: 37

Figure 6.24 Soon after surgery, the grade 2 hole has closed. The outer retina often closes last with a small cyst under the retina in the initial stages.

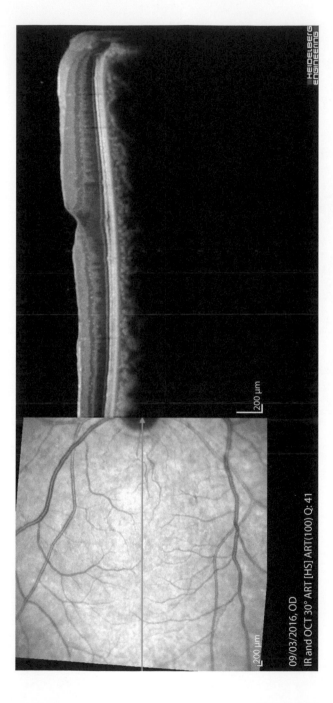

09/03/2016, OD

IR and OCT 30° ART [HS] ART(100) Q: 41

Figure 6.25 Closure of the grade 2 hole post-operatively and full resolution of the cyst. The good ellipsoid line is associated with high visual acuity.

Table 6.1 Macular hole

Condition	Characteristics	Referral	Why?
Macular hole	Duration: <12 months	Refer routinely if access is good (4–6 weeks)	Good surgical results
	Duration: >12 months	Discuss poor prognosis and refer if requested	Poor surgical results

scan. Vitreomacular traction syndrome is often accompanied by ERM, indicated by the attachment of the ERM to the posterior hyaloid membrane. The membrane is usually associated with the presence of mild CMO on fundus fluorescein angiography (FFA). Cavities in the retina can be seen on OCT and are an indication of damage to the retina from the action of the ERM. Occasionally, an ERM is seen without separation of the vitreous (Figures 6.26 through 6.31).[47]

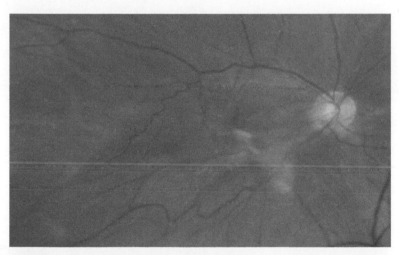

Figure 6.26 ERM on the macula distorting the blood vessels.

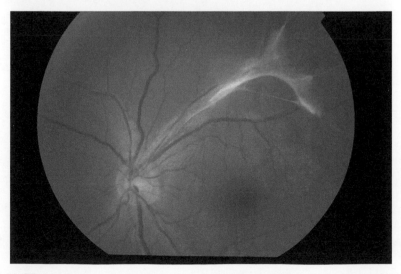

Figure 6.27 ERM on the vascular arcade is causing secondary wrinkling of the retina in the macula.

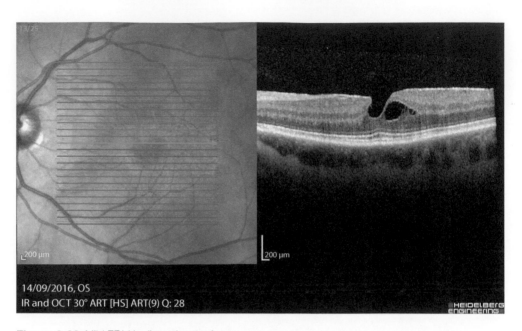

Figure 6.28 Mild ERM is disrupting the fovea.

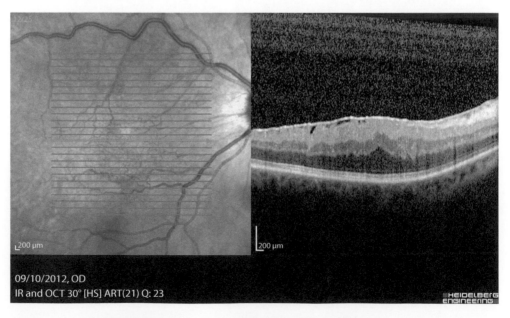

Figure 6.29 ERM has flattened out the retina causing loss of the foveal dip.

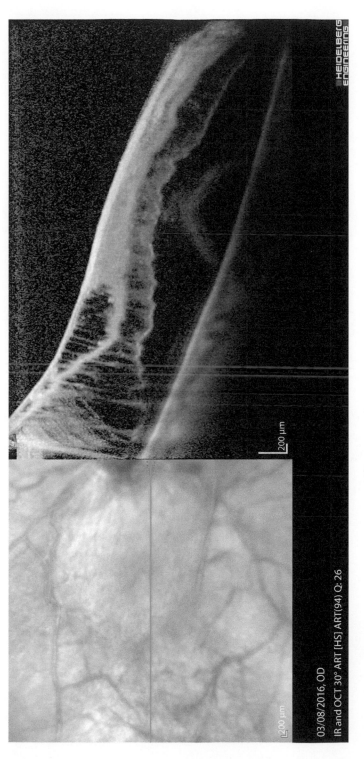

03/08/2016, OD

IR and OCT 30° ART [HS] ART(94) Q: 26

200 μm

200 μm

Figure 6.30 Severe ERM causes schisis of the retina and SRF under the fovea.

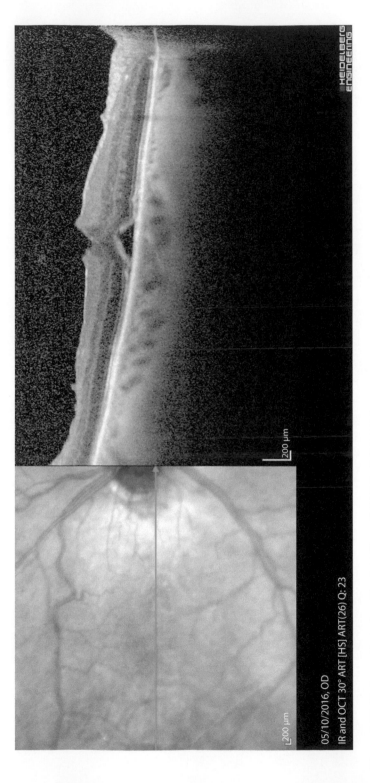

Figure 6.31 Post-operatively, the retina from Figure 6.30 is much improved.

Young patients usually have an attached vitreous gel. These patients may show a spontaneous separation of the ERM where the vitreous separates and peels the ERM off the retinal surface.[48]

OTHER CONDITIONS

Mild vitreous shrinkage with a taut posterior hyaloid membrane that is still attached to the retina may be partly responsible for cystoid macular oedema (CMO) in diabetic maculopathy or uveitis.

SECONDARY MACULAR PUCKER

ERM can be associated with the following:

- Retinal tear or retinal detachment[49]: 7%[50] of RRD but more common in PVR with a 6-month prevalence of 15%[51] and higher rates in post-mortem studies.[52] The ERM in RRD can occur rapidly with symptoms deteriorating over weeks.[53] Histologically, the ERM is more often associated with pigmented cells (RPE)[54] rather than microglial cells.
- BRVO, in which case, it is worth checking an FFA to assess the perifoveal arcade. If this is not complete, this may indicate a poorer prognosis for vision post-operatively.
- Posterior uveitis (Figure 6.32).
- Peripheral retinal angiomata, e.g. von Hippel–Lindau disease or idiopathic acquired angiomata.[55,56]
- Sickle cell disease in 4%.[57]
- Candida endophthalmitis.[58]
- Combined hamartoma of the disc in young patients.
- Familial exudative vitreoretinopathy (FEVR) in young patients (Figure 6.33).[59]

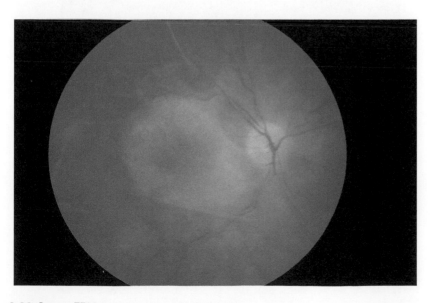

Figure 6.32 Severe ERM secondary to uveitis in the eye.

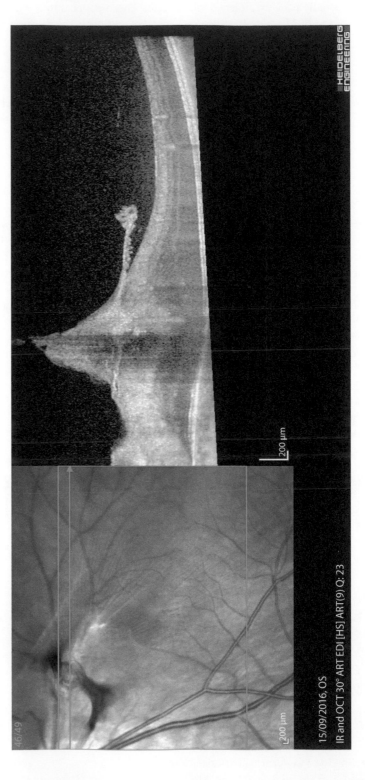

15/09/2016, OS

IR and OCT 30° ART EDI [HS] ART(9) Q: 23

Figure 6.33 ERM can be secondary to other conditions, e.g. in this case, from the rare condition of FEVR.

SUCCESS RATES OF SURGERY

The aim of surgery is to reduce distortion and improve visual acuity. Patients find distortion visually disabling. This has a better chance of improvement after surgery than visual acuity. Visual acuity can be improved in 80–86%[60,61] and to 20/60 or better in 75%. Two lines of improvement in acuity can be expected in those that respond to surgery.[62] Those with shorter duration, better presenting vision, thinner membranes and no retinal elevation do better.[63] Even if vision does not improve, the quality of life scores are improved after surgery probably because of the resolution or reduction of distortion, which is not generally measured by objective psychometric testing (Figures 6.34 through 6.37).[64]

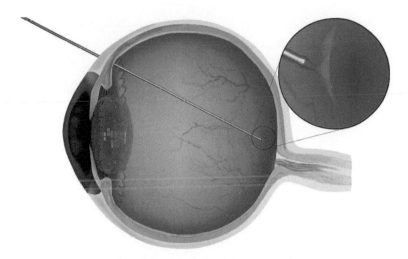

Figure 6.34 PPV is used to remove the vitreous. This allows the surgeon to gain access to the posterior segment. It is safer to manipulate instruments in a water-filled cavity rather than in a gel and collagen matrix (vitreous).

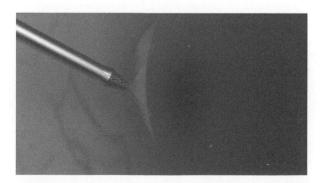

Figure 6.35 Once the vitreous is removed, the retina can be accessed for grasping the ERM for removal.

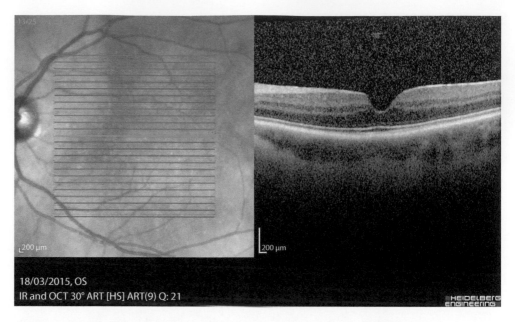

18/03/2015, OS
IR and OCT 30° ART [HS] ART(9) Q: 21

Figure 6.36 Eye with ERM has been operated upon, and the anatomy, much improved post-operatively.

SPECIFIC COMPLICATIONS OF SURGERY

- Cataract appears in 47–80%.[65,66] Surgeons may combine PPV with phacoemulsification cataract surgery.
- Damage to the ILM and nerve fibre layer occurs.[67,68]
- Persistent cystoid macular oedema can be seen, which is not responsive to intravitreal steroid or topical non-steroidal anti-inflammatory agents.
- Myopic post-operative refraction after cataract surgery may occur because the elevation of the retina in the macula by an ERM may lead to a short axial length during biometry and the use of an overly powerful intraocular lens.[69]
- Retinal tear and retinal detachment[70] occurs in 2.5%.[71] If PVD is created during surgery, retinal tears can occur in 32.1% compared to 2.1% in those without the induction of PVD.[72]

MEMBRANE RECURRENCE

This has been shown to occur in 4–20% of cases[73–75] but will respond to repeated surgery. The removal of the ILM during surgery has been reported to reduce recurrence rates.[75] Recurrence appears to be more common in secondary ERM, e.g. with retinal angiomata (30%)[76] and uveitis.[77]

REFERRAL

Referral of these cases is not so dependent on time. Most ERM develop within 9 months after a PVD. If a patient gives a good history of PVD and the ERM is detected within the first year

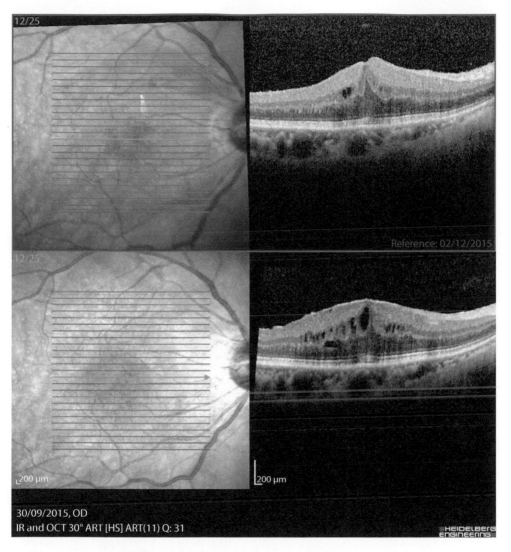

Figure 6.37 Thickening of the retina by ERM (pre-operatively: bottom) will not always be resolved after surgery (post-operative: top).

after PVD, observe the ERM for progression or refer promptly if they are symptomatic and want to be considered for surgery. Most ERMs do not present like this, however, and are seen without a history of PVD and are found to be stable. Most will be asymptomatic and not require referral. Those that are reducing vision or distorting the visual image can be referred routinely.

It is uncertain whether old ERMs will do less well than more recent ones, and it can be surprising how well long-standing ERM can respond to surgery. Therefore, surgery can be offered to all. Unpredictably and rarely, a stable ERM will change and progress, causing further reduction in vision (Figures 6.38 and 6.39) (Table 6.2).

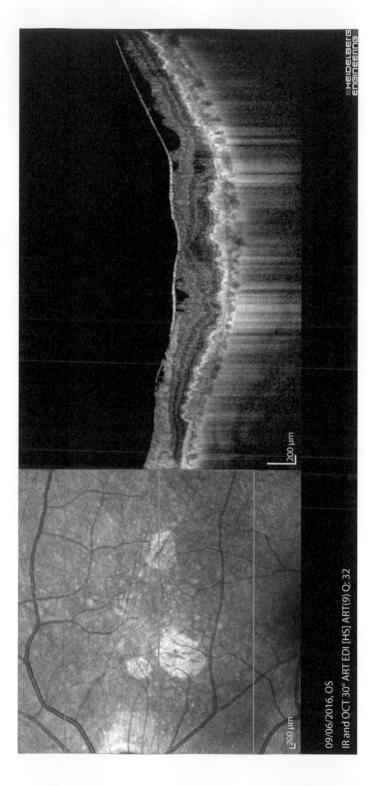

09/06/2016, OS

IR and OCT 30° ART EDI [HS] ART(9) Q: 32

200 μm

200 μm

Figure 6.38 Surgeries on eyes with AMD may show poorer vision despite successful removal of ERM.

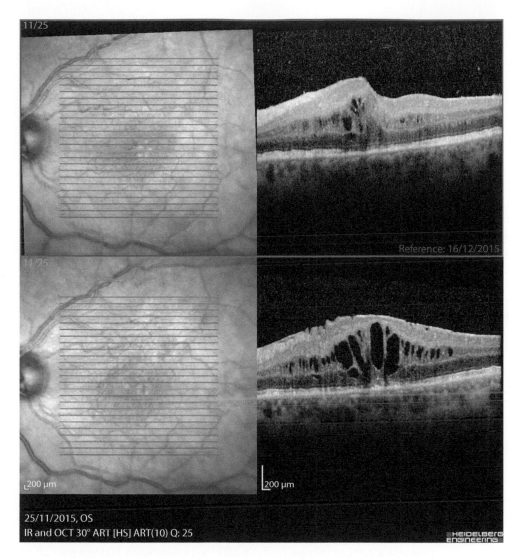

Figure 6.39 ERM can cause cavities in the retina. Some are from fluid leakage, but others are signs of damage to the retina and will not be resolved after surgery (post-operative image on the top).

Table 6.2 Macular ERM

Condition	Characteristics	Referral	Why?
Macular ERM	Duration: <24 months	Refer routinely (1–2 months)	Good surgical results
	Duration: >24 months	Discuss poor prognosis and refer if requested	Poor surgical results

AGE-RELATED MACULAR DEGENERATION

CLINICAL FEATURES

AMD can be classified as dry and wet macular degenerations.

Features of dry AMD include the following:

- Hard drusen
- Soft drusen
- Retinal pigment epithelial disruption
- Geographic atrophy

Patients with extensive small drusen, non-extensive intermediate size drusen or pigment abnormalities have only a 1.3% 5-year probability of progression to advanced AMD according to the age-related eye disease study (AREDS).[78] Those with extensive intermediate size drusen, at least one large drusen, non-central geographic atrophy in one or both eyes or advanced AMD or vision loss due to AMD in one eye are at risk of vision loss from advanced AMD in up to 50% (large drusen with pigmentary changes) after 5 years.[79] In wet AMD, there is fluid leakage in or under the retina from pigment epithelial detachment or choroidal neovascular membranes. Choroidal neovascular membranes are vascular membranes that commence in the choroid and penetrate the retinal layers.

SIMPLIFIED AREDS SCORING SYSTEM

- One or more large drusen (≥125 μm, width of a large vein at disc margin) in an eye = one risk factor
- Any pigment abnormality in an eye = one risk factor
- Risk factors summed across both eyes
- The 5-year risk of developing advanced AMD in at least one eye
  - 0 factor: 0.5%
  - 1 factor: 3%
  - 2 factors: 12%
  - 3 factors: 25%
  - 4 factors: 50%
- If no large drusen but intermediate drusen present in both eyes = one risk factor

This risk of progression has been shown by the AREDS to be reduced by taking a cocktail of high-dose vitamins (commercially available in combination preparations) with 500 mg vitamin C, 400 IU vitamin E, 15 mg beta-carotene (to be avoided by smokers or ex-smokers of less than 10 years because of an increased risk of lung carcinoma), 80 mg zinc, as zinc oxide, and 2 mg copper, as cupric oxide.[80] This cocktail may reduce the chance of advancement in patients with high-risk characteristics by approximately 30%.

Patients with choroidal neovascular membranes already in one eye are at particular risk of progressing to 'wet' ARMD with choroidal neovascular membranes production. The choroidal neovascular membranes cause distortion and loss of vision with serous elevation of the retina, subretinal haemorrhage and, finally, disciform scar formation.

Choroidal neovascular membranes are usually classified on fluorescein angiography into the following:

- Classic, dye leakage appearing early, located beneath the neuroretina
- Non-classic, indistinct and slower appearance of dye, located under the RPE
- Mixed, predominantly classic or non-classic

Table 6.3 Intravitreal injections for choroidal neovascularisation

Drug	Structure	Dosage	Route of administration
Ranibizumab (Lucentis)[83–85]	Antibody fragment; anti-VEGF	0.5 mg/0.05 mL	Intravitreal
Bevacizumab (Avastin)	Complete immunoglobulin; anti-VEGF	1.25 mg/0.05 mL	Intravitreal
Aflibercept (Eylea)	Antibody fragment; VEGF trap	2 mg/0.05 mL	Intravitreal

The frequent bilaterality of the condition results in a high proportion of patients who are technically blind, with severe loss of central vision. For this reason, surgical approaches have been tried in the past. However, these have largely been superseded by anti-vascular endothelial growth factor (anti-VEGF) treatments, bevacizumab,[81] aflibercept[82] and ranibizumab (Table 6.3).[83–85] The last two are now established as the therapies of choice for choroidal neovascular membranes from AMD.

Vitreomacular traction is more common in eyes with exudative AMD (38%) compared with non-exudative AMD (10%) and PVD less common (21% and 68%, respectively), suggesting to some investigators a role for the vitreous in exudative AMD.[86]

Vitrectomy surgery may be employed for the following:

- VH with choroidal neovascular membranes and subretinal haemorrhage
- Pneumatic displacement of subretinal haemorrhage
- Failure of anti-VEGF regimes

VITREOUS HAEMORRHAGE AND CHOROIDAL NEOVASCULAR MEMBRANES

A patient with sudden onset VH in the presence of a large subretinal craggy mass on ultrasound is very likely to have suffered a subretinal bleed from a choroidal neovascular membrane from AMD (Table 6.4).[87] The subretinal haemorrhage is usually in the macular area; occasionally, it is due to a peripheral choroidal neovascular membrane, and the macula is clear of blood. Removing the VH is useful for restoring peripheral vision, but the patient must be warned about the likelihood for reduced central vision. The haemorrhage is often very thick and may be altered to an ochre colour seen in severe bleeds. The vitreous may or may not be detached.

Often, these patients are on anti-platelet or anti-coagulation therapy.[88] The other eye may have evidence of AMD because the condition is usually bilateral.

REFERRAL

Sudden severe loss of vision in a patient with AMD may be from VH. Refer urgently because an ultrasound is required to confirm the diagnosis. Surgery is then required in a non-urgent manner to restore peripheral vision.

Table 6.4 VH and choroidal neovascular membranes

Condition	Characteristics	Referral	Why?
VH and choroidal neovascular membranes	Sudden loss of vision	Refer urgently	For ultrasound and diagnosis

PNEUMATIC DISPLACEMENT OF SUBRETINAL HAEMORRHAGE

A bleed from a choroidal neovascular membrane may spread under the macula, giving a rise to a large central scotoma (Table 6.5). It is possible to facilitate the resorption of the haemorrhage and perhaps to displace the bleed away from the fovea by performing PPV and gas, but this has to be done within the first 2 weeks; otherwise, the clot becomes organised and will not disperse. The patient is required to posture upright to allow the gas bubble to act on the haemorrhage, displacing it inferiorly. Either intravitreal tissue plasminogen activator (tPA) (0.05 mL, 50 µg) or subretinal tPA can be injected to facilitate the breakup of the clot (Figures 6.40 through 6.42).[89–92]

Table 6.5 Subretinal haemorrhage from choroidal neovascular membranes

Condition	Characteristics	Referral	Why?
Subretinal haemorrhage from choroidal neovascular membranes	Sudden loss of vision	Refer urgently	Vision improved by early surgery

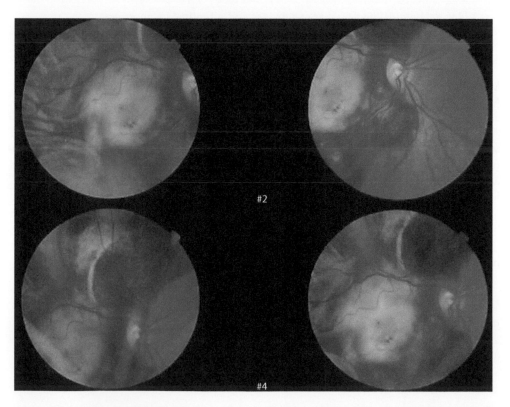

Figure 6.40 Large subretinal haemorrhage from a choroidal neovascular membrane. Systemic use of anti-platelet or anti-coagulant medications by the patient increases the risk of this complication.

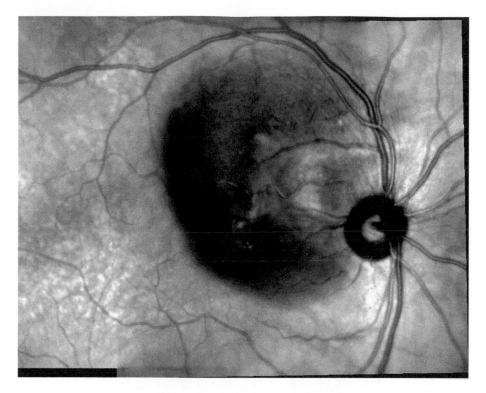

Figure 6.41 Subretinal haemorrhage from a peripapillary choroidal neovascular membrane.

REFERRAL

If you see a patient with a fresh subretinal bleed in the macula associated with AMD, it is worth referring urgently for an opinion. The pneumatic displacement of the blood appears to aid recovery of the vision if done within 2 weeks of onset.

CHOROIDAL NEOVASCULAR MEMBRANE NOT FROM AMD

INTRODUCTION

CNV can occur secondary to a variety of conditions. The choroidal neovascular membranes are often smaller and self-limiting. Surgical removal is possible with immediate restoration of vision or reduction in distortion but with a high chance of recurrence of approximately 30%; however, intravitreal injections are more likely to be employed.

Presumed ocular histoplasmosis[93–95] (also called punctate inner choroidopathy or multifocal inner choroidopathy in some countries), uveitis, choroidal rupture from trauma,[96] juxtafoveolar telangiectasia,[97] central serous chorioretinopathy[98] or macular surgery[99] can all be associated with choroidal neovascular membranes.[100] Angioid streaks and myopia[101–103] may produce choroidal neovascular membranes, but surgical removal is less successful. These are more likely to be treated by anti-VEGF therapies, but the membranes can be surgically removed with some success.

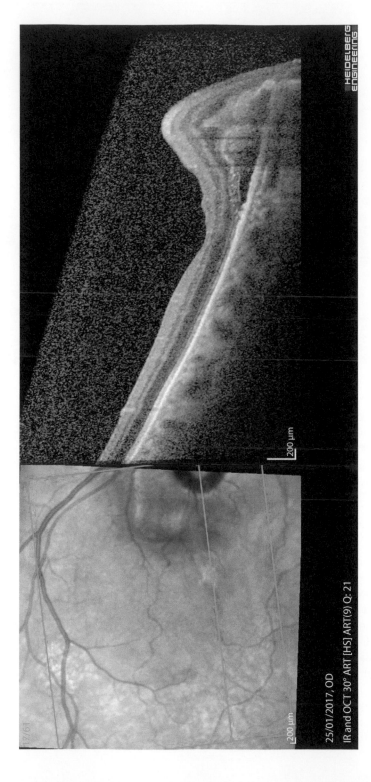

25/01/2017, OD

IR and OCT 30° ART [HS] ART(9) Q: 21

Figure 6.42 Subretinal injection of tissue plasminogen has been used to break up the blood clot with an intravitreal gas bubble to displace the haemorrhage away from the fovea. After surgery the vision has returned to 20/15.

REFERENCES

1. McCannel, C. A., Ensminger, J. L., Diehl, N. N. and Hodge, D. N. Population-based incidence of macular holes. *Ophthalmology* 2009;116(7):1366–9.

2. Lewis, M. L., Cohen, S. M., Smiddy, W. E. and Gass, J. D. Bilaterality of idiopathic macular holes. *Graefes Arch Clin Exp Ophthalmol* 1996;234(4):241–5.

3. Watzke, R. C. and Allen, L. Subjective slitbeam sign for macular disease. *Am J Ophthalmol* 1969;68(3):449–53.

4. Tanner, V. and Williamson, T. H. Watzke–Allen slit beam test in macular holes confirmed by optical coherence tomography. *Arch Ophthalmol* 2000;118(8):1059–63.

5. Ezra, E., Fariss, R. N., Possin, D. E. et al. Immunocytochemical characterization of macular hole opercula. *Arch Ophthalmol* 2001;119(2):223–31.

6. Ezra, E., Munro, P. M., Charteris, D. G. et al. Macular hole opercula: Ultrastructural features and clinicopathological correlation. *Arch Ophthalmol* 1997;115(11):1381–7.

7. Haouchine, B., Massin, P. and Gaudric, A. Foveal pseudocyst as the first step in macular hole formation: A prospective study by optical coherence tomography. *Ophthalmology* 2001;108(1):15–22.

8. Gass, J. D. Idiopathic senile macular hole: Its early stages and pathogenesis. *Arch Ophthalmol* 1988;106(5):629–39.

9. Gass, J. D. Reappraisal of biomicroscopic classification of stages of development of a macular hole. *Am J Ophthalmol* 1995;119(6):752–9.

10. Johnson, R. N. and Gass, J. D. Idiopathic macular holes: Observations, stages of formation, and implications for surgical intervention. *Ophthalmology* 1988;95(7):917–24.

11. Wakely, L., Rahman, R. and Stephenson, J. A comparison of several methods of macular hole measurement using optical coherence tomography, and their value in predicting anatomical and visual outcomes. *Br J Ophthalmol* 2012;96(7):1003–7.

12. de Bustros, S. Vitrectomy for prevention of macular holes: Results of a randomized multicenter clinical trial: Vitrectomy for Prevention of Macular Hole Study Group. *Ophthalmology* 1994;101(6):1055–9.

13. Kokame, G. T. and de Bustros, S. Visual acuity as a prognostic indicator in stage I macular holes: The Vitrectomy for Prevention of Macular Hole Study Group. *Am J Ophthalmol* 1995;120(1):112–4.

14. Kim, J. W., Freeman, W. R., el-Haig, W. et al. Baseline characteristics, natural history, and risk factors to progression in eyes with stage 2 macular holes: Results from a prospective randomized clinical trial: Vitrectomy for Macular Hole Study Group. *Ophthalmology* 1995;102(12):1818–28.

15. Ezra, E. and Gregor, Z. J. Surgery for idiopathic full-thickness macular hole: Two-year results of a randomized clinical trial comparing natural history, vitrectomy, and vitrectomy plus autologous serum: Morfields Macular Hole Study Group Report no. 1. *Arch Ophthalmol* 2004;122(2):224–36.

16. Freeman, W. R., Azen, S. P., Kim, J. W. et al. Vitrectomy for the treatment of full-thickness stage 3 or 4 macular holes: Results of a multicentered randomized clinical trial: The Vitrectomy for Treatment of Macular Hole Study Group. *Arch Ophthalmol* 1997;115(1):11–21.

17. Casuso, L. A., Scott, I. U., Flynn, H. W. Jr. et al. Long-term follow-up of unoperated macular holes. *Ophthalmology* 2001;108(6):1150–5.

18. Hee, M. R., Izatt, J. A., Swanson, E. A. et al. Optical coherence tomography of the human retina. *Arch Ophthalmol* 1995;113(3):325–32.

19. Tanner, V., Chauhan, D. S., Jackson, T. L. and Williamson, T. H. Optical coherence tomography of the vitreoretinal interface in macular hole formation. *Br J Ophthalmol* 2001;85(9):1092–7.
20. Chauhan, D. S., Antcliff, R. J., Rai, P. A. et al. Papillofoveal traction in macular hole formation: The role of optical coherence tomography. *Arch Ophthalmol* 2000;118(1):32–8.
21. Ito, Y., Terasaki, H., Suzuki, T. et al. Mapping posterior vitreous detachment by optical coherence tomography in eyes with idiopathic macular hole. *Am J Ophthalmol* 2003; 135(3):351–5.
22. Smiddy, W. E., Michels, R. G., de Bustros, S. et al. Histopathology of tissue removed during vitrectomy for impending idiopathic macular holes. *Am J Ophthalmol* 1989;108(4): 360–4.
23. Chan, A., Duker, J. S., Schuman, J. S. and Fujimoto, J. G. Stage 0 macular holes: Observations by optical coherence tomography. *Ophthalmology* 2004;111(11):2027–32.
24. Ismail, R., Tanner, V. and Williamson, T. H. Optical coherence tomography imaging of severe commotio retinae and associated macular hole. *Br J Ophthalmol* 2002;86(4):473–4.
25. Yamashita, T., Uemara, A., Uchino, E. et al. Spontaneous closure of traumatic macular hole. *Am J Ophthalmol* 2002;133(2):230–5.
26. Chen, Y. P., Chen, T. L., Chao, A. N. et al. Surgical management of traumatic macular hole-related retinal detachment. *Am J Ophthalmol* 2005;140(2):331–3.
27. Sakaguchi, H., Ohji, M., Kubota, A. et al. Amsler grid examination and optical coherence tomography of a macular hole caused by accidental Nd:YAG laser injury. *Am J Ophthalmol* 2000;130(3):355–6.
28. Spaide, R. F. Closure of an outer lamellar macular hole by vitrectomy: Hypothesis for one mechanism of macular hole formation. *Retina* 2000;20(6):587–90.
29. Haouchine, B., Massin, P., Tadayoni, R. et al. Diagnosis of macular pseudoholes and lamellar macular holes by optical coherence tomography. *Am J Ophthalmol* 2004;138(5):732–9.
30. Patel, B., Duvall, J. and Tullo, A. B. Lamellar macular hole associated with idiopathic juxtafoveolar telangiectasia. *Br J Ophthalmol* 1988;72(7):550–1.
31. Unoki, N., Nishijima, K., Kita, M. et al. Lamellar Macular Hole Formation in Patients with Diabetic Cystoid Macular Edema. *Retina* 2009.
32. Gass, J. D. Lamellar macular hole: A complication of cystoid macular edema after cataract extraction. *Arch Ophthalmol* 1976;94(5):793–800.
33. Hirakawa, M., Uemura, A., Nakano, T. and Sakamoto, T. Pars plana vitrectomy with gas tamponade for lamellar macular holes. *Am J Ophthalmol* 2005;140(6):1154–5.
34. Garretson, B. R., Pollack, J. S., Ruby, A. J. et al. Vitrectomy for a symptomatic lamellar macular hole. *Ophthalmology* 2008;115(5):884–6.
35. de Smet, M. D., Gandorfer, A., Stalmans, P. et al. Microplasmin intravitreal administration in patients with vitreomacular traction scheduled for vitrectomy: The MIVI I trial. *Ophthalmology* 2009;116(7):1349–55, 55.
36. Haynes, R. J., Yorston, D., Laidlaw, D. A. et al. Real world outcomes of ocriplasmin use by members of the British and Eire Association of Vitreoretinal Surgeons. *Eye (Lond)* 2017;31(1):107–12.
37. Williamson, T. H. and Lee, E. Idiopathic macular hole: Analysis of visual outcomes and the use of indocyanine green or brilliant blue for internal limiting membrane peel. *Graefes Arch Clin Exp Ophthalmol* 2014;252(3):395–400.
38. Michalewska, Z., Michalewski, J., Adelman, R. A. and Nawrocki, J. Inverted internal limiting membrane flap technique for large macular holes. *Ophthalmology* 2010;117(10): 2018–25.

39. Messmer, E. M., Heidenkummer, H. P. and Kampik, A. Ultrastructure of epiretinal membranes associated with macular holes. *Graefes Arch Clin Exp Ophthalmol* 1998; 236(4):248–54.

40. Snead, D. R, Cullen, N., James, S. et al. Hyperconvolution of the inner limiting membrane in vitreomaculopathies. *Graefes Arch Clin Exp Ophthalmol* 2004;242(10):853–62.

41. De Juan, E. Jr., Lambert, H. M. and Machemer, R. Recurrent proliferations in macular pucker, diabetic retinopathy, and retrolental fibroplasialike disease after vitrectomy. *Graefes Arch Clin Exp Ophthalmol* 1985;223(4):174–83.

42. Smiddy, W. E., Michels, R. G., Gilbert, H. D. and Green, W. R. Clinicopathologic study of idiopathic macular pucker in children and young adults. *Retina* 1992;12(3):232–6.

43. Ng, C. H., Cheung, N., Wang, J. J. et al. Prevalence and risk factors for epiretinal membranes in a multi-ethnic United States population. *Ophthalmology* 2011;118(4):694–9.

44. Klein, R., Klein, B. E., Wang, Q. and Moss, S. E. The epidemiology of epiretinal membranes. *Trans Am Ophthalmol Soc* 1994;92:403–25; discussion 25–30.

45. Allen, A. W. Jr. and Gass, J. D. Contraction of a perifoveal epiretinal membrane simulating a macular hole. *Am J Ophthalmol* 1976;82(5):684–91.

46. Martinez, J., Smiddy, W. E., Kim, J. and Gass, J. D. Differentiating macular holes from macular pseudoholes. *Am J Ophthalmol* 1994;117(6):762–7.

47. Meyer, C. H., Rodrigues, E. B., Mennel, S. et al. Spontaneous separation of epiretinal membrane in young subjects: Personal observations and review of the literature. *Graefes Arch Clin Exp Ophthalmol* 2004;242(12):977–85.

48. Desatnik, H., Treister, G. and Moisseiev, J. Spontaneous separation of an idiopathic macular pucker in a young girl. *Am J Ophthalmol* 1999;127(6):729–31.

49. de Bustros, S., Rice, T. A., Michels, R. G. et al. Vitrectomy for macular pucker: Use after treatment of retinal tears or retinal detachment. *Arch Ophthalmol* 1988;106(6):758–60.

50. Lobes, L. A. Jr. and Burton, T. C. The incidence of macular pucker after retinal detachment surgery. *Am J Ophthalmol* 1978;85(1):72–7.

51. Cox, M. S., Azen, S. P., Barr, C. C. et al. Macular pucker after successful surgery for proliferative vitreoretinopathy: Silicone Study Report 8. *Ophthalmology* 1995;102(12):1884–91.

52. Wilson, D. J. and Green, W. R. Histopathologic study of the effect of retinal detachment surgery on 49 eyes obtained post mortem. *Am J Ophthalmol* 1987;103(2):167–79.

53. Sheard, R. M., Sethi, C. and Gregor, Z. Acute macular pucker. *Ophthalmology* 2003; 110(6):1178–84.

54. Cherfan, G. M., Smiddy, W. E., Michels, R. G. et al. Clinicopathologic correlation of pigmented epiretinal membranes. *Am J Ophthalmol* 1988;106(5):536–45.

55. Laatikainen, L., Immonen, I. and Summanen, P. Peripheral retinal angiomalike lesion and macular pucker. *Am J Ophthalmol* 1989;108(5):563–6.

56. Machemer, R. Peripheral retinal angiomalike lesion and macular pucker. *Am J Ophthalmol* 1990;109(2):244.

57. Carney, M. D. and Jampol, L. M. Epiretinal membranes in sickle cell retinopathy. *Arch Ophthalmol* 1987;105(2):214–7.

58. McDonald, H. R., de Bustros, S. and Sipperley, J. O. Vitrectomy for epiretinal membrane with Candida chorioretinitis. *Ophthalmology* 1990;97(4):466–9.

59. Mason, J. O. III and Kleiner, R. Combined hamartoma of the retina and retinal pigment epithelium associated with epiretinal membrane and macular hole. *Retina* 1997; 17(2):160–2.

60. Trese, M. T., Chandler, D. B. and Machemer, R. Macular pucker: I. Prognostic criteria. *Graefes Arch Clin Exp Ophthalmol* 1983;221(1):12–5.
61. Haritoglou, C., Gandorfer, A., Gass, C. A. et al. The effect of indocyanine-green on functional outcome of macular pucker surgery. *Am J Ophthalmol* 2003;135(3):328–37.
62. Dawson, S. R., Shunmugam, M. and Williamson, T. H. Visual acuity outcomes following surgery for idiopathic epiretinal membrane: An analysis of data from 2001 to 2011. *Eye (Lond)* 2014;28(2):219–24.
63. de Bustros, S., Thompson, J. T., Michels, R. G. et al. Vitrectomy for idiopathic epiretinal membranes causing macular pucker. *Br J Ophthalmol* 1988;72(9):692–5.
64. Ghazi-Nouri, S. M., Tranos, P. G., Rubin, G. S. et al. Visual function and quality of life following vitrectomy and epiretinal membrane peel surgery. *Br J Ophthalmol* 2006;90(5):559–62.
65. Cherfan, G. M., Michels, R. G., de Bustros, S. et al. Nuclear sclerotic cataract after vitrectomy for idiopathic epiretinal membranes causing macular pucker. *Am J Ophthalmol* 1991;111(4):434–8.
66. de Bustros, S., Thompson, J. T., Michels, R. G. et al. Nuclear sclerosis after vitrectomy for idiopathic epiretinal membranes. *Am J Ophthalmol* 1988;105(2):160–4.
67. Maguire, A. M., Smiddy, W. E., Nanda, S. K. et al. Clinicopathologic correlation of recurrent epiretinal membranes after previous surgical removal. *Retina* 1990;10(3):213–22.
68. Trese, M., Chandler, D. B. and Machemer, R. Macular pucker: II. Ultrastructure. *Graefes Arch Clin Exp Ophthalmol* 1983;221(1):16–26.
69. Manvikar, S., Steel, D. and Pimenidis, D. Refractive outcome of phacovitrectomy. *J Cataract Refract Surg* 2008;34(12):2009–10.
70. Michels, R. G. and Gilbert, H. D. Surgical management of macular pucker after retinal reattachment surgery. *Am J Ophthalmol* 1979;88(5):925–9.
71. Guillaubey, A., Malvitte, L., Lafontaine, P. O. et al. Incidence of retinal detachment after macular surgery: A retrospective study of 634 cases. *Br J Ophthalmol* 2007;91(10):1327–30.
72. Chung, S. E., Kim, K. H. and Kang, S. W. Retinal breaks associated with the induction of posterior vitreous detachment. *Am J Ophthalmol* 2009;147(6):1012–6.
73. Michels, R. G. Vitrectomy for macular pucker. *Ophthalmology* 1984;91(11):1384–8.
74. Grewing, R. and Mester, U. Results of surgery for epiretinal membranes and their recurrences. *Br J Ophthalmol* 1996;80(4):323–6.
75. Park, D. W., Dugel, P. U., Garda, J. et al. Macular pucker removal with and without internal limiting membrane peeling: Pilot study. *Ophthalmology* 2003;110(1):62–4.
76. McDonald, H. R., Schatz, H., Johnson, R. N. et al. Vitrectomy in eyes with peripheral retinal angioma associated with traction macular detachment. *Ophthalmology* 1996;103(2):329–35.
77. Verbraeken, H. Therapeutic pars plana vitrectomy for chronic uveitis: A retrospective study of the long-term results. *Graefes Arch Clin Exp Ophthalmol* 1996;234(5):288–93.
78. Harooni, M., McMillan, T. and Refojo, M. Efficacy and safety of enzymatic posterior vitreous detachment by intravitreal injection of hyaluronidase. *Retina* 1998;18(1):16–22.
79. Ferris, F. L., Davis, M. D., Clemons, T. E. et al. A simplified severity scale for age-related macular degeneration: AREDS Report No. 18. *Arch Ophthalmol* 2005;123(11):1570–4.
80. Age-related eye disease research study group. A randomized, placebo-controlled, clinical trial of high-dose supplementation with vitamins C and E, beta carotene, and zinc for age-related macular degeneration and vision loss: AREDS report no. 8. *Arch Ophthalmol* 2001;119(10):1417–36.
81. Avery, R. L., Pieramici, D. J., Rabena, M. D. et al. Intravitreal bevacizumab (Avastin) for neovascular age-related macular degeneration. *Ophthalmology* 2006;113(3):363–72.

82. Schmidt-Erfurth, U., Kaiser, P. K., Korobelnik, J. F. et al. Intravitreal aflibercept injection for neovascular age-related macular degeneration: Ninety-six-week results of the VIEW studies. *Ophthalmology* 2014;121(1):193–201.

83. Rosenfeld, P. J., Rich, R. M. and Lalwani, G. A. Ranibizumab: Phase III clinical trial results. *Ophthalmol Clin North Am* 2006;19(3):361–72.

84. Rosenfeld, P. J., Brown, D. M., Heier, J. S. et al. Ranibizumab for neovascular age-related macular degeneration. *N Engl J Med* 2006;355(14):1419–31.

85. Brown, D. M., Kaiser, P. K., Michels, M. et al. Ranibizumab versus verteporfin for neovascular age-related macular degeneration. *N Engl J Med* 2006;355(14):1432–44.

86. Robison, C. D., Krebs, I., Binder, S. et al. Vitreomacular adhesion in active and end-stage age-related macular degeneration. *Am J Ophthalmol* 2009;148(1):79–82 e2.

87. Orth, D. H. and Flood, T. P. Management of breakthrough vitreous hemorrhage from presumed extramacular subretinal neovascularization. *Retina* 1982;2(2):89–93.

88. Kuhli-Hattenbach, C., Fischer, I. B., Schalnus, R. and Hattenbach, L. O. Subretinal hemorrhages associated with age-related macular degeneration in patients receiving anticoagulation or antiplatelet therapy. *Am J Ophthalmol* 2007;149(2):316–21 e1.

89. Gopalakrishan, M., Giridhar, A., Bhat, S. et al. Pneumatic displacement of submacular hemorrhage: Safety, efficacy, and patient selection. *Retina* 2007;27(3):329–34.

90. Ohji, M., Saito, Y., Hayashi, A. et al. Pneumatic displacement of subretinal hemorrhage without tissue plasminogen activator. *Arch Ophthalmol* 1998;116(10):1326–32.

91. Hesse, L., Meitinger, D. and Schmidt, J. Little effect of tissue plasminogen activator in subretinal surgery for acute hemorrhage in age-related macular degeneration. *Ger J Ophthalmol* 1996;5(6):479–83.

92. Singh, R. P., Patel, C. and Sears, J. E. Management of subretinal macular haemorrhage by direct administration of tissue plasminogen activator. *Br J Ophthalmol* 2006;90(4):429–31.

93. Atebara, N. H., Thomas, M. A., Holekamp, N. M. et al. Surgical removal of extensive peripapillary choroidal neovascularization associated with presumed ocular histoplasmosis syndrome. *Ophthalmology* 1998;105(9):1598–605.

94. Melberg, N. S., Thomas, M. A., Dickinson, J. D. and Valluri, S. Managing recurrent neovascularization after subfoveal surgery in presumed ocular histoplasmosis syndrome. *Ophthalmology* 1996;103(7):1064–7.

95. Lit, E. S., Kim, R. Y. and Damico, D. J. Surgical removal of subfoveal choroidal neovascularization without removal of posterior hyaloid: A consecutive series in younger patients. *Retina* 2001;21(4):317–23.

96. Gross, J. G., King, L. P., De Juan, E. Jr. and Powers, T. Subfoveal neovascular membrane removal in patients with traumatic choroidal rupture. *Ophthalmology* 1996;103(4):579–85.

97. Berger, A. S., McCuen, B. W., Brown, G. C. and Brownlow, R. L. Jr. Surgical removal of subfoveal neovascularization in idiopathic juxtafoveolar retinal telangiectasis. *Retina* 1997;17(2):94–8.

98. Cooper, B. A. and Thomas, M. A. Submacular surgery to remove choroidal neovascularization associated with central serous chorioretinopathy. *Am J Ophthalmol* 2000;130(2):187–91.

99. Ng, E. W., Bressler, N. M., Boyer, D. S. and De Juan, E. Jr. Iatrogenic choroidal neovascularization occurring in patients undergoing macular surgery. *Retina* 2002;22(6):711–8.

100. Hawkins, B. S., Miskala, P. H., Bass, E. B. et al. Surgical removal vs observation for subfoveal choroidal neovascularization, either associated with the ocular histoplasmosis syndrome or idiopathic: II. Quality-of-life findings from a randomized clinical trial: SST Group H Trial: SST Report No. 10. *Arch Ophthalmol* 2004;122(11):1616–28.

101. Ruiz-Moreno, J. M. and de la Vega, C. Surgical removal of subfoveal choroidal neovascularisation in highly myopic patients. *Br J Ophthalmol* 2001;85(9):1041–3.
102. Uemura, A. and Thomas, M. A. Subretinal surgery for choroidal neovascularization in patients with high myopia. *Arch Ophthalmol* 2000;118(3):344–50.
103. Uemura, A. and Thomas, M. A. Visual outcome after surgical removal of choroidal neovascularization in pediatric patients. *Arch Ophthalmol* 2000;118(10):1373–8.

Diabetic retinopathy

INTRODUCTION

There are a number of conditions that stimulate new blood vessel formation (neovascularisation [NV]) of the retina. These blood vessels are fragile, risking VH and associated with fibrosis and contraction causing tractional retinal detachment (TRD). The most common condition is severe diabetic retinopathy; others are retinal vein occlusion (RVO), sickle cell retinopathy and retinal vasculitis.

DIABETIC RETINOPATHY

INTRODUCTION

Despite major advances in screening of the diabetic population in some countries and improved clinical management of patients, the surgical complications of diabetic retinopathy are on the increase because the proportion of the population with type 2 diabetes is increasing. Retinal laser photocoagulation is the mainstay of therapy[1–3] and reduces the chance of sight loss by 50%. Vitrectomy is performed for VH or TRD with a 5% vitrectomy rate in diabetic retinopathy for over 5 years.[4] There is increased recording of the use of PPV with endolaser photocoagulation by 86% in Medicare fee data from the United States from 1997 to 2007.[5] In the same period, the application of laser was stable. Rates of progression to vitrectomy are reduced by good control of blood sugar, hypertension and lipids and timely and early panretinal photocoagulation (PRP), which reduced the risk of PPV to 2.3% from 4% in the early treatment diabetic retinopathy study (ETDRS).[6] The prevalence of PPV in the diabetic population in south London, UK, has been estimated as 5:1000 diabetic patients.

DIABETIC RETINOPATHY GRADING

Ischaemic diabetic retinopathy characteristically affects the midperipheral retina, as seen on fluorescein angiography (Table 7.1). NV develops near the posterior limit of the ischaemia, i.e. at the optic disc and along the major vascular arcades. The vascular tissue arises from intraretinal venules and proliferates within the most cortical part of the vitreous gel as a vascularised ERM. The vessels do not grow into the central gel except occasionally within Cloquet's canal. The membranes

Table 7.1 Diabetic retinopathy grading

Grade	Retinal features
No diabetic retinopathy	Nil
Mild non-proliferative retinopathy (NPDR)	Microaneurysms only
Moderate NPDR	More than 'microaneurysms only' and less than severe NPDR
Severe NPDR	Any of the following: • More than 20 microaneurysms in each quadrant • Venous beading in more than two quadrants • Intraretinal microvascular abnormalities in more than one quadrant • No proliferation
Proliferative	Low risk, flat new vessels elsewhere High risk, raised new vessels elsewhere or disc new vessels

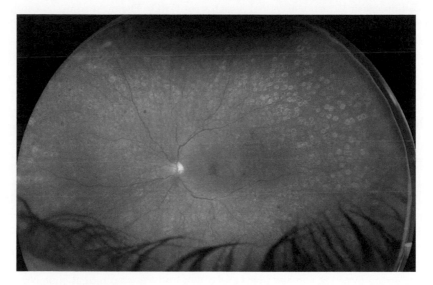

Figure 7.1 PRP in a diabetic patient.

incarcerate the gel, resulting in adhesion between the retina and the vitreous. The vitreous may stiffen and shrink secondarily to the retinopathy, increasing the traction on blood vessels and membranes. The vitreous may detach from the retina rupturing blood vessels (Figure 7.1).

DIABETIC VITREOUS HAEMORRHAGE

The diabetic retinopathy study (DRS), and ETDRS, examining the use of laser therapy in diabetic retinopathy showed reduction in sight loss by 50–70%[6–8] (Table 7.2).

Table 7.2 Baseline demographic information in south London, United Kingdom

Demographics	
Male	54.1%
Type 1	36.8%
Type 2	63.2%
Insulin requiring	71.4%
Ethnicity	
Afro-Caribbean	31.4%
Caucasian	53.5%
South east Asian	11.4%

CLINICAL FEATURES

This is the most common cause of haemorrhage into the vitreous. Haemorrhage may occur into the gel, retrohyaloid space or, rarely, subretinal space (the last usually in association with TRD and associated with a poor visual outcome[9]). Severe retrohyaloid haemorrhage may cause the posterior vitreous face to bulge forward into bullae, looking slightly like retinal detachment to the unwary. Often, diabetic haemorrhaging occurs spontaneously, i.e. from action of the vitreous on the new blood vessels, but occasionally, haemorrhage happens during vigorous isometric exertion, which raises the systemic blood pressure. Approximately 50% of the haemorrhages will clear spontaneously over 3 months, but in most circumstances, surgery is the better choice than observation because untreated NV may progress over this time, risking further haemorrhage, TRD or neovascular glaucoma. Type 1 diabetics are particularly at risk of further complications if left too long before surgery.[10,11] While waiting for clearance, it is important to monitor the IOP for erythroclastic glaucoma and to perform repeated ultrasound examinations for retinal detachment (Table 7.3).

Causes of VH are as follows:

- Active neovascularisation (NV)
- Inactive NV
- Vessel avulsion
- Traction from vitreous
- Pathological shrinkage of the vitreous
- Mobility of the vitreous
- PVD
- Acutely raised BP (Figure 7.2)

Table 7.3 When to do more PRP and when to perform PPV in patients with diabetic VH

PRP	PPV
Active NV and view rapidly clearing	Non-clearing VH duration 2–3/12
	Inadequate PRP
	Iris NV
	For visual rehabilitation

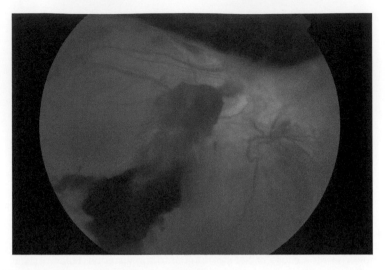

Figure 7.2 There is not only VH but also underlying TRD.

The indicators for early surgical intervention are as follows:

- Iris NV: urgent
- No previous PRP: urgent
- Erythroclastic glaucoma: soon
- Type 1 diabetes: soon

B scan ultrasound examination is important to determine where the blood is situated, whether there is TRD, RRD or PVD, and is accurate in 90% of cases.[12] The adhesion of the vitreous to the retina can be seen on the ultrasound at the sites of neovascularisation often on the vascular arcades or at the optic disc. The role of vitrectomy in the management of the complications of diabetic retinopathy has been established for many years.[13–15] The success rates of PPV are now high enough to offer surgery early in the clinical course of the haemorrhage.

In some circumstances, if the VH is mild, further laser can be applied to try to regress the NV without PPV. Some patients will bleed despite extensive PRP because of the presence of established NV, which, although fibrosed, may haemorrhage from traction from the gel. These patients will not respond to further laser and will require PPV. The role of anti-VEGF injections in the treatment of VH is uncertain, although claims of more rapid regression of haemorrhage with injection have been made.[16]

Although VH from DMR may clear spontaneously after some months, PPV is frequently required to rehabilitate the patient and can be associated with better visual prognosis.[17]

If the optical media are clear, subhyaloid blood can sometimes be treated with yttrium aluminium garnet laser[18,19] without the need for vitrectomy. The haemorrhage spreads into the vitreous gel and clears from there. Vitrectomy may be a more reliable method however (Table 7.4).

Table 7.4 Referral for diabetic complications vitreous haemorrhage

Condition	Characteristics	Referral	Why?
Diabetic	VH with PRP	Routine referral of 1–2 months	Low risk of progression as the retina has been treated
	VH without PRP	2–3 weeks	There is a high risk of progression

DIABETIC RETINAL DETACHMENT

CLINICAL FEATURES

As in other ERMs, fibroblasts within the vascularised membranes contract and produce fibrosis (collagen synthesis). The contraction of the neovascular membranes both anteroposteriorly and tangentially combined with the shrinkage of the vitreous gel pulls the retina centrally. The retina detaches with a concave configuration as the RPE counteracts the traction on the retina (Figures 7.3 and 7.4).

The areas of detachment surround NV on the retinal arcades and are often multifocal. Eventually, the macula detaches severely reducing the visual acuity (VA), while the periphery remains flat. The extent of TRD varies from a single focus to large areas of the retina (Figures 7.5 through 7.7)

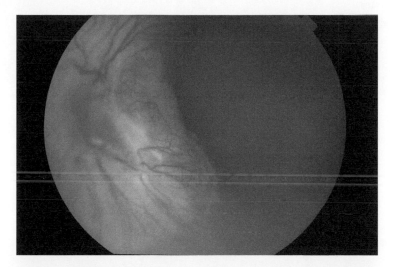

Figure 7.3 Neovascular component of the diabetic membranes is illustrated in this eye.

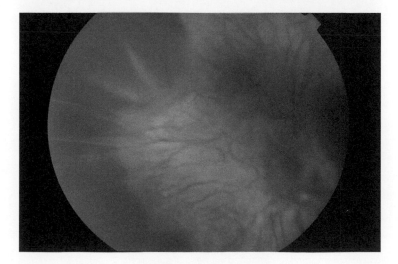

Figure 7.4 Severe TRD of the eye involving the macula.

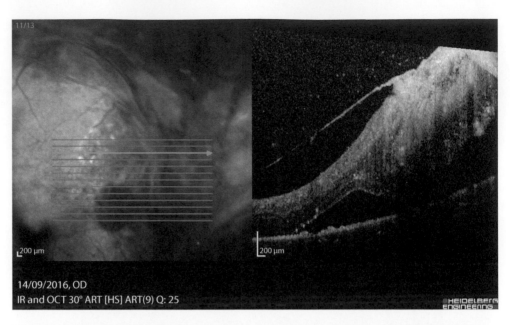

Figure 7.5 Retina is being detached from traction from contraction of fibrosed neovascular complexes.

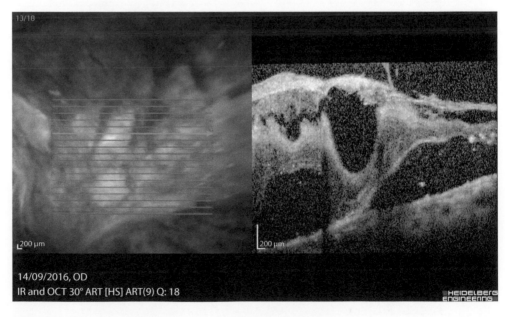

Figure 7.6 Retina and membrane are attached via pegs of adhesion.

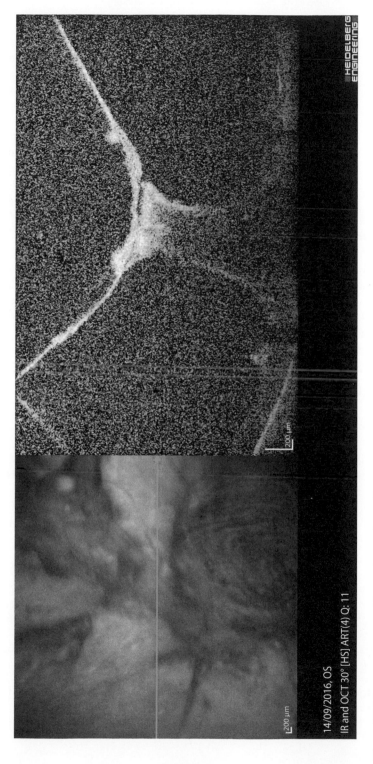

14/09/2016, OS

IR and OCT 30° [HS] ART(4) Q: 11

Figure 7.7 Vitreous contracts adding to the tractional effect on the retina.

Table 7.5 Referral for diabetic tractional retinal detachment

Condition	Characteristics	Referral	Why?
Diabetic	TRD with the macula recently detached	Emergency or urgent depending on duration of fovea off	Need to reattach the fovea quickly
	TRD with PRP macula on	Routine referral	If stable, may not need surgery
	TRD without PRP; macula on	1–2 weeks	Active NV risks progression of the RD
	Combined RRD/TRD	Emergency or urgent	Depends on the duration particularly the fovea

Traction on the disc can reduce vision by damaging the superficial nerve fibres[20]; indeed, axons are found in tissue removed from the disc surgically.[21]

Traction on the retina may split the retina causing retinoschisis.[21]

Occasionally, a hole appears in the fragile ischaemic retina allowing SRF accumulation. The retinal detachment then takes on a convex configuration and may extend further anteriorly in a bullous fashion. The application of PRP to eyes with TRD can cause further contraction of the membranes and macular detachment.[22] Therefore, in patients with established TRDs but with no PRPs it is often safer to perform PPV (Table 7.5).

SUCCESS RATES

For visual improvement

- VH: 90%
  - The Diabetic Retinopathy Vitrectomy Study (DRVS) from the 1980s included group 1, patients with recent severe VH (VA ≤ 5/200). Patients were randomised to PPV in 3 months or 1 year.[23] The chance of at least 10/20 was 25% in the early PPV patients and 15% in late PPV. The chance of no perception of light (NPL) was 25% with the early PPV and 19% in late PPV (not statistically significant).
  - Most benefit was found for early PPV in type 1 diabetics.
- TRD: 60% chance of improving the vision.
  - 50% achieving 20/200 or better,[24] 86% flat retina; recurrent TRD has been described in 22% and RRD in 7%.
  - DRVS group 2 included advanced proliferative diabetic retinopathy and vision at least 10/200 randomised to PPV or conventional management. The chance of VA at least 10/20 was 44% in the PPV group compared to 28%.
- Combined TRD/RRD: Chance of improved vision is approximately 50%.

The risk of NPL after PPV for diabetic retinopathy is 7%, increased in those patients with peroperative iris NV, or post-operative haemorrhage, macular ischaemia or iris NV.[25] Overall the reoperation rate is 16% (Figure 7.8).[25]

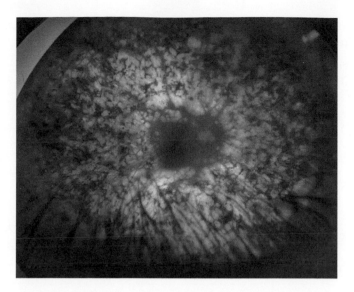

Figure 7.8 Severe diabetic retinopathy extensive laser is required to control the process. The laser burns grow slowly in size over time, and a small area of central retina may be all that remains functionally.

DIABETIC MACULOPATHY

This is the major cause of visual loss in type 2 diabetes and is therefore present in many patients undergoing vitrectomy.[26] Many investigations have been performed to investigate the role of vitrectomy in diabetic macular oedema.[27] [38] Randomised controlled trials without the addition of cataract surgery have shown no benefit.[39] PPV appears to normalise retinal microcirculation from its hyperdynamic pre-operative state.[40] A specific presentation of taut thickened posterior hyaloid membrane where a contraction of the vitreous is seen as a diffuse area of traction on the macula appears to respond to surgery probably because the diabetic maculopathy associated with this condition is much less.[41]

Macular holes (foveal) can very occasionally appear in the diabetic macula.[22]

The removal of massive subretinal exudation has been performed but is of uncertain worth,[42–44] and the drainage of fluid from cystoid spaces via retinal puncture has been attempted but again is not an established therapy.[45]

RETINAL VEIN OCCLUSION

RVOs are the second commonest vascular events in the eye after diabetic retinopathy. The eye is unusual in suffering from occlusion of the veins more often than arteries. RVO can be divided into two groups, BRVO and CRVO (including hemiretinal vein occlusion). BRVO occurs most commonly where a retinal arteriole and a venule cross each other perhaps because the thickened arteriolar wall compresses the thinner-walled venule, resulting in occlusion. In CRVO, the site of obstruction is situated at the lamina cribrosa.[46] A number of vitreoretinal innovations have been designed, but none are of proven benefit.

- Chorioretinal anastomosis: CRVO
- PPV: CRVO and BRVO
- Arteriovenous decompression: BRVO
- Radial optic neurotomy: CRVO
- TPA: CRVO

Anti-VEGF agents have been used widely for cystoid macular oedema from many causes, including RVO with low complication rates, but require repeat injection over a prolonged period. Anti-VEGF agents are also useful for controlling neovascular glaucoma.

SICKLE CELL DISEASE

INTRODUCTION

The sickle cell haemoglobinopathies result from an abnormality in the beta chain of the haemoglobin molecule. They are hereditary disorders that cause RBCs to take on a sickle shape in hypoxic or acidotic conditions. In this form, the blood cells are rigid and pass with more difficulty through blood vessels, causing vascular occlusion in multiple organs including the retina. There is chronic haemolytic anaemia and vaso-occlusive crises can occur. It produces a variety of clinical features in the eye.[47]

TYPES OF SICKLE CELL DISEASE

- Sickle cell trait (Hb AS)
- Sickle cell anaemia, homozygous sickle cell disease (SS disease)
- Sickle cell disease, heterozygous sickle cell C disease (SC disease)
- Sickle cell thalassaemia disease (S-thal disease)

SYSTEMIC INVESTIGATION

Ask for a history of systemic crisis, medications, racial and family history and check haemoglobin electrophoresis and full blood count (Figure 7.9).

INHERITANCE AND RACE

It is an autosomal, incomplete dominant condition (inheritance is similar to recessive inheritance, e.g. one in four chances of SS if both parents are AS), but the S gene can have effects if combined with the C gene or thalassaemia gene.

The sickle gene is present in approximately 8% of the African population in the United States but can be higher or lower depending on geographical location. The gene is thought to have originated in West Africa and become more prevalent because of its protective effect in falciparum malaria (shorter living RBCs and relative hypoxia may be detrimental to the infection). The gene is also seen in eastern Mediterranean and Middle Eastern patients. Patients with SC disease develop more retinal complications; however, complications are also seen in

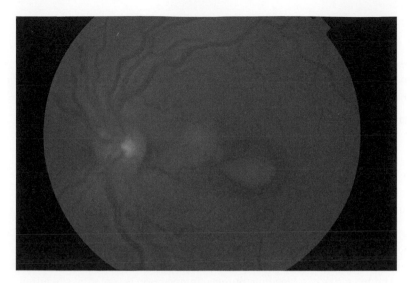

Figure 7.9 Pre-retinal haemorrhage in a patient with sickle cell disease.

SS disease. Most cases of retinopathy appear in patients between 20 and 40 years of age and stabilise or regress thereafter.

SYSTEMIC MANIFESTATIONS

- Painful vaso-occlusive crisis
- Acute chest crisis
- Anaemia
- Leg ulcers
- Bacterial infections
- Arthritis and swelling in the hands and feet
- Bone necrosis
- Splenomegaly
- Hepatomegaly
- Heart and lung damage

OPHTHALMIC PRESENTATION

The sickle blood cells occlude the retinal blood vessel causing hypoxia and stimulating NV. These may bleed or fibrose and contract, producing traction on the retina. The contraction may create retinal breaks and retinal detachment. The process also causes secondary changes in the vitreous, which stimulate macular ERM formation and macular holes. Retinal complications are seen in 43% of patients aged between 20 and 30 years with sickle cell.[48] In one study, blindness in patients with PVR was seen in 12%.[49] However, in a large study of young patients in Jamaica (307 patients with SS and 166 with SC disease), followed for 20 years up to the age of 26 years, only two patients had sight-threatening disease, one patient suffering irreversible sight loss in one eye and one patient with a successfully treated RRD.[48] A description of the natural history of the condition had VH in 5.3% and macular lesions in 4.6% and a low risk of retinal detachment in 2% over a mean follow-up of 6.3 years.[47]

The asymptomatic patient has the following:

- Black sunburst spots in the retina
- Iridescent spots in the retina
- Retinal haemorrhages (salmon patches)
- Sea fan neovascular proliferation

The symptomatic patient has the following[50]:

- VH
- TRD
- RRD
- Macular ERM
- Macular hole

The conjunctival and optic nerve head blood vessels show segmentation of blood columns in the homozygous sickle cell disease (SS). There may be comma-shaped vessels on the bulbar conjunctiva and iris atrophy from ischaemia. Spontaneous hyphaema can occur and cause raised IOP and has a risk of rebleeding. Surgical intervention is sometimes required.

The optic nerve may show dark red spots or clumps on the surface.

- Macula
  - Chronic retinal ischaemia
  - Macular ERM
  - Macular hole
  - Association with angioid streaks has been described
- Peripheral retina (Figure 7.10)
  - Non-proliferative changes
  - Venous tortuosity
  - Salmon patch haemorrhage: round or oval intraretinal haemorrhages in the midperiphery, initially bright red then fading to the colour of salmon flesh
  - Black sunburst: hypertrophy of the RPE with spiky border (Figure 7.11)
  - Iridescent white spots

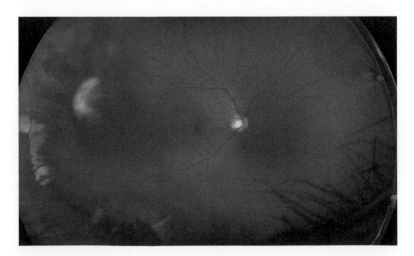

Figure 7.10 Sickle cell retinopathy peripheral retinal changes.

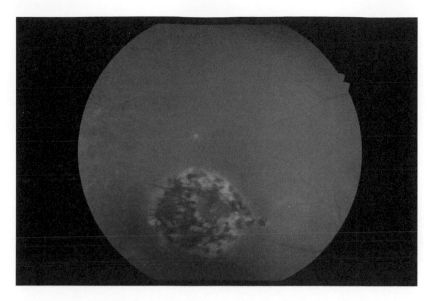

Figure 7.11 Black sunburst lesion in sickle cell.

- Proliferative changes, for which the Goldberg classification can be used[51]
- Peripheral arteriolar occlusion in the far periphery
- Arteriolar venular anastomosis seen at the junction of the perfused and non-perfused retina; best seen on angiography, flat on the retina and non-leaking
- Neovascular proliferation in the far periphery giving a 'sea fan' appearance; these often autoinfarct and are most common in SC disease; once infracted, a white fibrous scar remains
- VH
- Retinal detachment either tractional or rhegmatogenous (Figures 7.12 and 7.13)

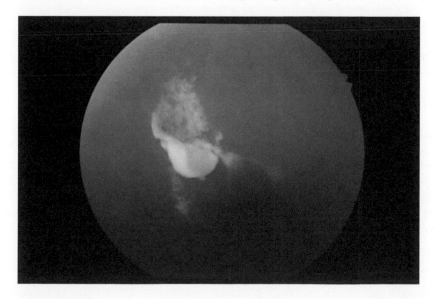

Figure 7.12 Sickle sea fan.

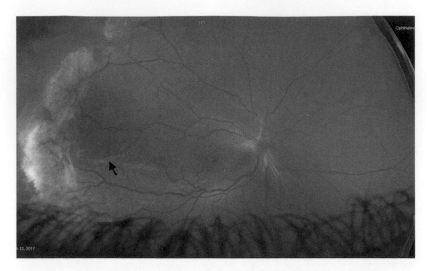

Figure 7.13 RRD in a patient with sickle retinopathy. The arrow indicates the retinal break.

VISUAL OUTCOME

In general, the risk to vision is low, and most complications are responsive to surgery. After the age of 40 years, the condition usually stabilises. In one study, outcomes for visions were good with 10 of 18 eyes achieving 20/40 vision or better and 15 eyes (83%) with improved vision after vitreoretinal surgery.[52]

SCREENING

The need for surveillance is doubtful because of the following:

- There is doubt over the effectiveness of prophylactic therapy, e.g. scatter laser (in contrast to diabetic retinopathy where it is of proven benefit).
- There is a relatively low prevalence of sight-threatening complications.
- Sight-threatening complications present symptomatically and usually progress slowly.
- Sight-threatening complications respond well to surgery if necessary.[53]

SURVIVAL

- Sickle cell anaemia (homozygous SS): The median age at death is 42 years for males and 48 years for females.[54]
- Sickle cell haemoglobin SC disease: The median age at death is 60 years for males and 68 years for females.
- 18% of the deaths occur in patients from organ failure, usually renal.
- 33% die during an acute sickle crisis (78% had pain, chest syndrome or both; 22% had stroke).

RETINAL VASCULITIS

In patients with retinal vasculitis, retinal NV can occur and cause VH or TRD. The former can be surgically removed, but care is required because vitreoretinal adhesions are common. PRP can be applied, and an increase in immunosuppressive cover may help the new vessels to regress. TRD tends to be associated with severe subretinal exudation and cholesterol crystal formation. The dissection of traction membranes is difficult and visual recovery is frequently poor.

CENTRAL RETINAL ARTERY OCCLUSION

In investigational surgery, the embolus in the central retinal artery occlusion has been surgically removed by incising the wall of the artery over the embolus.[55] The embolus exits the artery spontaneously or by grasping the embolus with forceps. Only a few patients have been described, and the technique has not become established because the patients would require the treatment within a few hours of the onset of the occlusion.

MEDICOLEGAL CASE

A diabetic patient is under review for pre-proliferative diabetic retinopathy. The patient is observed over the years until some retinal neovascularisation is detected, on which laser PRP is applied. The patient is carefully monitored every few months.

Fibrosis of the new vessels causes some degree of TRD. There is a gap in the follow-up for 1 year when the patient is unable to attend the service. The vision drops during this period, and when the patient is seen again, there is TRD spreading through the fovea of one eye. The patient is referred urgently for consideration of vitrectomy surgery on the eye.

A vitrectomy is performed. Post-operatively there are problems with persistent retinal detachment and raised IOP. Finally, the vision is lost in that eye.

On diagnosis of the pre-retinal fibrosis and TRD, there was a period when the patient was not seen. This was associated with the progression of TRD. Referral of the patient for consideration for surgery was prompt and cannot be criticized. The surgery was unsuccessful in repairing the retinal detachment, but this was a complex surgery with a known failure rate.

The reasons for the gap in the care of the patient would need to be elucidated but might have been from poor attendance from the patient. The delay might have contributed to the poorer outcome from surgery.

REFERENCES

1. Larsson, L. and Osterlin, S. Posterior vitreous detachment: A combined clinical and physiochemical study. *Graefes Arch Clin Exp Ophthalmol* 1985;223(2):92–5.
2. Walton, K. A., Meyer, C. H., Harkrider, C. J. et al. Age-related changes in vitreous mobility as measured by video B scan ultrasound. *Exp Eye Res* 2002;74(2):173–80.
3. Kado, M., Jalkh, A. E., Yoshida, A. et al. Vitreous changes and macular edema in central retinal vein occlusion. *Ophthalmic Surg* 1990;21(8):544–9.
4. Flynn, H. W. Jr., Chew, E. Y., Simons, B. D. et al. Pars plana vitrectomy in the Early Treatment Diabetic Retinopathy Study: ETDRS report number 17: The Early Treatment Diabetic Retinopathy Study Research Group. *Ophthalmology* 1992;99(9):1351–7.
5. Ramulu, P. Y., Do, D. V., Corcoran, K. J. et al. Use of retinal procedures in Medicare beneficiaries from 1997 to 2007. *Arch Ophthalmol* 2010;128(10):1335–40.

6. Early photocoagulation for diabetic retinopathy: ETDRS report number 9: Early Treatment Diabetic Retinopathy Study Research Group. *Ophthalmology* 1991;98(5 Suppl):766–85.

7. Photocoagulation treatment of proliferative diabetic retinopathy: The second report of diabetic retinopathy study findings. *Ophthalmology* 1978;85(1):82–106.

8. Photocoagulation treatment of proliferative diabetic retinopathy: Clinical application of Diabetic Retinopathy Study (DRS) findings, DRS Report Number 8: The Diabetic Retinopathy Study Research Group. *Ophthalmology* 1981;88(7):583–600.

9. Morse, L. S., Chapman, C. B., Eliott, D. et al. Subretinal hemorrhages in proliferative diabetic retinopathy. *Retina* 1997;17(2):87–93.

10. Sebag, J. Abnormalities of human vitreous structure in diabetes. *Graefes Arch Clin Exp Ophthalmol* 1993;231(5):257–60.

11. Akiba, J. Prevalence of posterior vitreous detachment in high myopia. *Ophthalmology* 1993;100(9):1384–8.

12. Genovesi-Ebert, F., Rizzo, S., Chiellini, S. et al. Reliability of standardized echography before vitreoretinal surgery for proliferative diabetic retinopathy. *Ophthalmologica* 1998;212 Suppl 1:91–2.

13. Mandelcorn, M. S., Blankenship, G. and Machemer, R. Pars plana vitrectomy for the management of severe diabetic retinopathy. *Am J Ophthalmol* 1976;81(5):561–70.

14. Michels, R. G. Vitrectomy for complications of diabetic retinopathy. *Arch Ophthalmol* 1978;96(2):237–46.

15. Aaberg, T. M. Clinical results in vitrectomy for diabetic traction retinal detachment. *Am J Ophthalmol* 1979;88(2):246–53.

16. Huang, Y. H., Yeh, P. T., Chen, M. S. et al. Intravitreal bevacizumab and panretinal photocoagulation for proliferative diabetic retinopathy associated with vitreous hemorrhage. *Retina* 2009;29(8):1134–40.

17. Yonemoto, J., Ideta, H., Sasaki, K. et al. The age of onset of posterior vitreous detachment. *Graefes Arch Clin Exp Ophthalmol* 1994;232(2):67–70.

18. Celebi, S. and Kukner, A. S. Photodisruptive Nd:YAG laser in the management of premacular subhyaloid hemorrhage. *Eur J Ophthalmol* 2001;11(3):281–6.

19. Ulbig, M. W., Mangouritsas, G., Rothbacher, H. H. et al. Long-term results after drainage of premacular subhyaloid hemorrhage into the vitreous with a pulsed Nd:YAG laser. *Arch Ophthalmol* 1998;116(11):1465–9.

20. Kroll, P., Wiegand, W. and Schmidt, J. Vitreopapillary traction in proliferative diabetic vitreoretinopathy [see comments]. *Br J Ophthalmol* 1999;83(3):261–4.

21. Pendergast, S. D., Martin, D. F., Proia, A. D. et al. Removal of optic disc stalks during diabetic vitrectomy. *Retina* 1995;15(1):25–8.

22. Ghoraba, H. Types of macular holes encountered during diabetic vitrectomy. *Retina* 2002;22(2):176–82.

23. Two-year course of visual acuity in severe proliferative diabetic retinopathy with conventional management: Diabetic Retinopathy Vitrectomy Study (DRVS) report #1. *Ophthalmology* 1985;92(4):492–502.

24. La Heij E. C., Tecim S., Kessels A. G. et al. Clinical variables and their relation to visual outcome after vitrectomy in eyes with diabetic retinal traction detachment. *Graefes Arch Clin Exp Ophthalmol* 2004;242(3):210–7.

25. Mason, J. O. III, Colagross, C. T., Haleman, T. et al. Visual outcome and risk factors for light perception and no light perception vision after vitrectomy for diabetic retinopathy. *Am J Ophthalmol* 2005;140(2):231–5.

26. Tong, L., Vernon, S. A., Kiel, W. et al. Association of macular involvement with prolif- erative retinopathy in Type 2 diabetes. *Diabet Med* 2001;18(5):388–94.

27. Kuhn, F., Kiss, G., Mester, V. et al. Vitrectomy with internal limiting membrane removal for clinically significant macular oedema. *Graefes Arch Clin Exp Ophthalmol* 2004; 242(5):402–8.

28. Micelli, F. T., Cardascia, N., Durante, G. et al. Pars plana vitrectomy in diabetic macular edema. *Doc Ophthalmol* 1999;97(3–4):471–4.

29. Ikeda, T., Sato, K., Katano, T. and Hayashi, Y. Vitrectomy for cystoid macular oedema with attached posterior hyaloid membrane in patients with diabetes. *Br J Ophthalmol* 1999;83(1):12–4.

30. Ikeda, T., Sato, K., Katano, T. and Hayashi, Y. Attached posterior hyaloid membrane and the pathogenesis of honeycombed cystoid macular edema in patients with diabetes. *Am J Ophthalmol* 1999;127(4):478–9.

31. Tachi, N. and Ogino, N. Vitrectomy for diffuse macular edema in cases of diabetic reti- nopathy. *Am J Ophthalmol* 1996;122(2):258–60.

32. Yamamoto, T., Hitani, K., Tsukahara, I. et al. Early postoperative retinal thickness changes and complications after vitrectomy for diabetic macular edema. *Am J Ophthalmol* 2003;135(1):14–9.

33. Harbour, J. W., Smiddy, W. E., Flynn, H. W. Jr. and Rubsamen, P. E. Vitrectomy for dia- betic macular edema associated with a thickened and taut posterior hyaloid membrane. *Am J Ophthalmol* 1996;121(4):405–13.

34. Pendergast, S. D., Hassan, T. S., Williams, G. A. et al. Vitrectomy for diffuse diabetic macular edema associated with a taut premacular posterior hyaloid. *Am J Ophthalmol* 2000;130(2):178–86.

35. La Heij, E. C., Hendrikse, F., Kessels, A. G. and Derhaag, P. J. Vitrectomy results in diabetic macular oedema without evident vitreomacular traction. *Graefes Arch Clin Exp Ophthalmol* 2001;239(4):264–70.

36. Sato, Y., Lee, Z. and Shimada, H. Vitrectomy for diabetic cystoid macular edema. *Jpn J Ophthalmol* 2002;46(3):315–22.

37. Otani, T. and Kishi, S. A controlled study of vitrectomy for diabetic macular edema. *Am J Ophthalmol* 2002;134(2):214–9.

38. Lewis, H., Abrams, G. W., Blumenkranz, M. S. and Campo, R. V. Vitrectomy for diabetic macular traction and edema associated with posterior hyaloidal traction. *Ophthalmology* 1992;99(5):753–9.

39. Thomas, D., Bunce, C., Moorman, C. and Laidlaw, D. A. A randomised controlled feasibility trial of vitrectomy versus laser for diabetic macular oedema. *Br J Ophthalmol* 2005;89(1):81–6.

40. Park, J. H., Woo, S. J., Ha, Y. J. and Yu, H. G. Effect of vitrectomy on macular microcircu- lation in patients with diffuse diabetic macular edema. *Graefes Arch Clin Exp Ophthalmol* 2009;247(8):1009–17.

41. Laidlaw, D. A. Vitrectomy for diabetic macular oedema. *Eye* 2008;22(10):1337–41.

42. Yang, C. M. Surgical treatment for severe diabetic macular edema with massive hard exudates. *Retina* 2000;20(2):121–5.

43. Sakuraba, T., Suzuki, Y., Mizutani, H. and Nakazawa, M. Visual improvement after removal of submacular exudates in patients with diabetic maculopathy. *Ophthalmic Surg Lasers Imaging Retina* 2000;31(4):287–91.

44. Takagi, H., Otani, A., Kiryu, J. and Ogura, Y. New surgical approach for removing mas- sive foveal hard exudates in diabetic macular edema. *Ophthalmology* 1999;106(2):249–56.

45. Singh, R. P., Margolis, R. and Kaiser, P. K. Cystoid puncture for chronic cystoid macular oedema. *Br J Ophthalmol* 2007;91(8):1062–4.

46. Green, W. R., Chan, C. C., Hutchins, G. M. and Terry, J. M. Central retinal vein occlusion: A prospective histopathologic study of 29 eyes in 28 cases. *Trans Am Ophthalmol Soc* 1981;79:371–422.

47. Clarkson, J. G. The ocular manifestations of sickle-cell disease: A prevalence and natural history study. *Trans Am Ophthalmol Soc* 1992;90:481–504.

48. Downes, S. M., Hambleton, I. R., Chuang, E. L. et al. Incidence and natural history of proliferative sickle cell retinopathy: Observations from a cohort study. *Ophthalmology* 2005;112(11):1869–75.

49. Condon, P., Jampol, L. M., Farber, M. D. et al. A randomized clinical trial of feeder vessel photocoagulation of proliferative sickle cell retinopathy. II. Update and analysis of risk factors. *Ophthalmology* 1984;91(12):1496–8.

50. Brazier, D. J., Gregor, Z. J., Blach, R. K. et al. Retinal detachment in patients with proliferative sickle cell retinopathy. *Trans Ophthalmol Soc UK* 1986;105 (Pt 1):100–5.

51. Goldberg, M. F. Classification and pathogenesis of proliferative sickle retinopathy. *Am J Ophthalmol* 1971;71(3):649–65.

52. Williamson, T. H., Rajput, R., Laidlaw, D. A. and Mokete, B. Vitreoretinal management of the complications of sickle cell retinopathy by observation or pars plana vitrectomy. *Eye (Lond)* 2009;23(6):1314–20.

53. Saidkasimova, S., Shalchi, Z., Mahroo, O. A. et al. Risk factors for visual impairment in patients with sickle cell disease in London. *Eur J Ophthalmol* 2016;26(5):431–5.

54. Platt, O. S., Brambilla, D. J., Rosse, W. F. et al. Mortality in sickle cell disease. Life expectancy and risk factors for early death. *N Engl J Med* 1994;330(23):1639–44.

55. Garcia-Arumi, J., Martinez-Castillo, V., Boixadera, A. et al. Surgical embolus removal in retinal artery occlusion. *Br J Ophthalmol* 2006;90(10):1252–5.

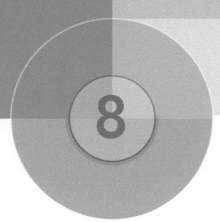

Trauma

INTRODUCTION

Ocular trauma remains a leading cause of visual loss internationally, most often affecting men (five males to one female). Patients are usually aged less than 30 years; trauma may be associated with alcohol and illicit drug usage.[1] Elderly males and females are more equally involved.[2] Incidence has been estimated as 3:10,000 of population.[3,4] Severe injuries, which might require vitreoretinal surgery, account for 5% of all eye injuries.[5] Aetiology is highly variable, but certain associations are common, e.g. assault; sport; children at play; road traffic accidents; and industrial, domestic and war injuries.[6–9] The patterns of ocular trauma are constantly changing depending on social, demographic and geographical variations. Intraocular foreign bodies (IOFBs) are common in war[9] and road traffic accidents, especially when car seat belts are not worn.[10] In children, sharp objects are commonly implicated, and the complication of amblyopia limits potential visual recovery.[11] The wearing of spectacles has been found to be relatively protective.[12]

CLASSIFICATION

The Birmingham Eye Trauma Terminology System can be used to describe these cases[13]:

1. Eye wall: sclera and cornea
2. Closed globe injury: no full-thickness wound of eye wall
3. Open globe injury: full-thickness wound of the eye wall
4. Contusion: no (full-thickness) wound
5. Lamellar laceration: partial-thickness wound of the eye wall
6. Rupture: full-thickness wound of the eye wall, caused by a blunt object
7. Laceration: full-thickness wound of the eye wall, caused by a sharp object
8. Penetrating injury: entrance wound or wounds from object or objects
9. IOFB: intraocular foreign body in the eye
10. Perforating injury: entrance and exit wounds from the same object

The injury may involve the use of blunt objects as in assaults from fists, feet or wooden bats; from other causes, e.g. balls in sport, air bags,[14–16] paint balls[17] and bungee elastic cords[18]; or from sharp instruments such as broken glass, knives or fragments of metal.

Trauma was an early indication for the use of vitrectomy.[19–26]

CONTUSION INJURIES

CLINICAL PRESENTATION

- Presentations of contusion injury
  - Subluxated or dislocated lens
  - VH
  - Macular oedema and commotio retinae
  - Retinal detachment from
    - Dialysis usually with a 'bucket handle' vitreous base avulsion
    - GRT
    - Ragged retinal tear in an area of commotion retinae
    - Pars ciliaris tear
- Late retinal pigment epithelial changes
- Macular hole
- Choroidal rupture, haemorrhage
- Choroidal neovascular membrane
- Optic nerve avulsion

Contusion injuries occur when an object strikes the eye, but the eye wall remains intact. This is common in assaults from the use of fists or feet or from injury from balls in sport but can also be encountered from air bags,[14–16] paint balls[17] and bungee elastic cords.[18]

In mild injury, the retina shows commotio retina (whitening), sometimes accompanied by macular oedema (Berlin's oedema).

Vision can be lost from the following:

- Hyphaema
- Macular oedema
- Commotio retinae
- Choroidal rupture
- Lens dislocation
- Glaucoma
- Retinal detachment
- Choroidal haemorrhage
- VH
- Macular hole

Corneal staining can result from very severe hyphaema.

Choroidal neovascular membrane may complicate choroidal rupture.

The retina may show late retinal pigment epithelial changes from diffused retinal damage.

Lens dislocation may occur in patients with pseudoexfoliation or pseudophakia or in highly myopic eyes.

Ultrasound is helpful to assess the type of haemorrhage in patients with medial opacities to determine prognosis for vision and surgical options. Traumatic macular hole formation may occur.

TYPES OF RETINAL BREAK

DIALYSIS

In blunt trauma, the most common break is an inferotemporal dialysis with superonasal quadrant as the next most common (see Chapter 5).[27] The patient may not be symptomatic for some time because of the slow onset of detachment and late detachment of the macula. Occasionally, an avulsion of the vitreous base is seen comprising a strip of ciliary epithelium, ora serrata and immediately post-oral retina into which the basal vitreous gel remains inserted called a 'bucket handle'. Some patients can present with giant dialysis (90–360°) (Figures 8.1 through 8.4).

Refer as an emergency.

Figure 8.1 Retinal break at the ora serrata is called a dialysis. The vitreous is attached.

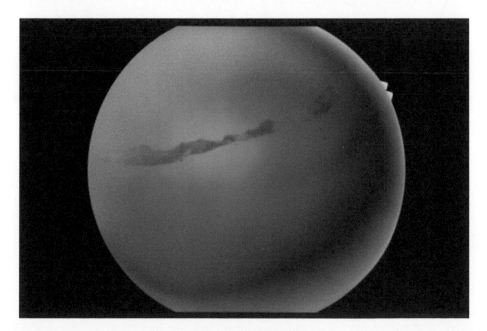

Figure 8.2 Bucket handle opacity from the vitreous base tearing away from the ora serrata in a patient with a blunt trauma and an underlying dialysis and retinal detachment.

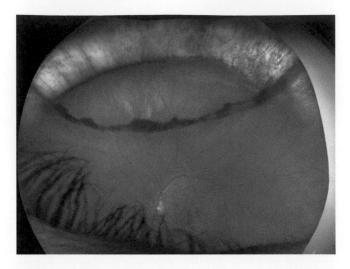

Figure 8.3 Bucket handle in the patient above after surgery. The indentation from the external buckle can be seen with a flat retina.

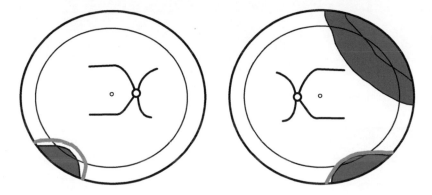

Figure 8.4 Drawing of a patient who had two inferior dialyses, which were stable and had a pigmented edge. He was then struck in the eye by a champagne cork and developed a further dialysis in the left eye superiorly.

PAR CILIARIS TEARS

In a few cases, retinal tears may be found in the non-pigmented epithelium of the pars ciliaris. These are rare and very difficult to detect, typically causing a slow-onset shallow retinal detachment.[28] This should be considered in children with a poor history of the onset of the retinal detachment and a chronic RRD.

Refer as an emergency.

RAGGED TEAR IN COMMOTIO RETINAE

In severe injury, the choroid and retina have an ischaemic and haemorrhagic appearance (scloptera) and can produce a ragged degenerative break that may be large. This should be

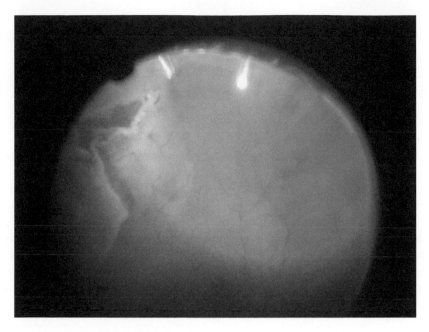

Figure 8.5 Ragged retinal break from trauma.

treated by observation at first, but these can cause retinal detachment and be associated with VH when intervention is indicated[29] (Figure 8.5).

Refer as an emergency.

GIANT RETINAL TEARS

PVD-related tears can be seen most often as GRTs, but they also appear occasionally as U tears. Refer as an emergency

PVR is a risk in a severely traumatised and haemorrhagic eye (for surgery, see Chapter 4).

Macular holes can be treated by surgery.

VISUAL OUTCOME

The visual outcome is dependent on the mechanism of injury, but contusion injury severe enough to require vitreoretinal intervention is associated with only a 50% chance of better than 20/200 vision (Table 8.1).

Table 8.1 Contusion

Condition	Characteristic	Referral	Why?
Trauma	Contusion	Emergency	Assessment is required to look for sight threatening complications

RUPTURE

CLINICAL PRESENTATION

Blunt trauma may rupture the eye wall, most commonly, the sclera at the limbus or posterior to the extraocular muscle insertions often with immediate loss of the crystalline lens and prolapse of the choroid and retina (Figure 8.6). Old surgical wounds are also prone to opening, e.g. corneal grafts and extracapsular cataract extraction wounds. Clinically recognising that a rupture has occurred is difficult and must be suspected in an injured eye with intraocular haemorrhage, vitreal or choroidal, after blunt trauma (Table 8.2).

In one study, 72% of eyes with severe blunt trauma had scleral ruptures; 47% of these were undetected pre-operatively.[30] Computed tomography (CT) cannot be relied upon to detect globe rupture.[31] The severe fibrotic response that trauma induces[32] leads to a high incidence of retinal detachment, which may progress rapidly to closed funnel detachments within weeks.

Surgical exploration of the globe may be required early on to clear extruded tissues from the wound and to allow wound closure. The incarceration of vitreous, choroid and retina into scleral ruptures cause traction on these structures and progressive incarceration of the tissues over time. This leads to total retinal detachment (Figures 8.7 and 8.8).

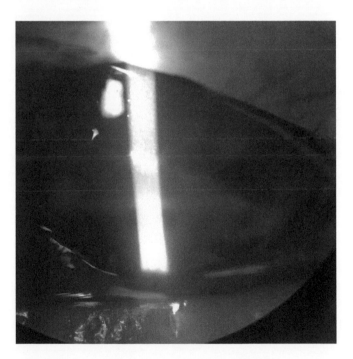

Figure 8.6 Severe hyphaema in a patient with choroidal haemorrhaging.

Table 8.2 Rupture

Condition	Characteristic	Referral	Why?
Trauma	Rupture	Emergency	Needs primary repair and antibiotics

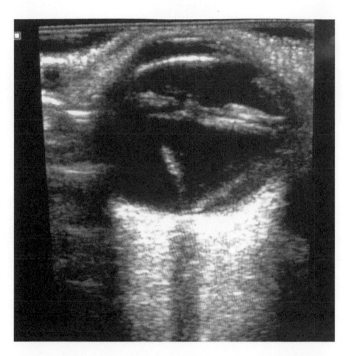

Figure 8.7 Golf ball struck this eye. There was a temporal scleral rupture. The ultrasound shows a contraction of the vitreous behind the lens, and there is a total retinal detachment.

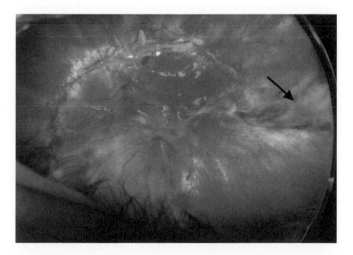

Figure 8.8 Three hundred sixty degree retinectomy has been performed on the retina, but there are persistent membranes and retinal detachment in this traumatised eye. The arrow indicates the site of the rupture of the globe.

In practice, if rupture is present, the posterior segment is often disrupted with choroidal and VH, and there is a deepened anterior chamber. Take care not to exacerbate the extrusion of intraocular contents by applying pressure to the globe during any examination.

The IOP in rupture may be normal or even high because the scleral rupture may block off with intraocular or orbital tissue.

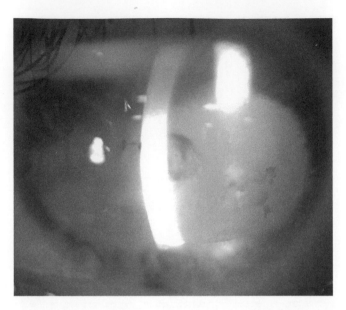

Figure 8.9 Band keratopathy is the calcification of the cornea and seen in oil-filled eyes after a number of years.

Ultrasound can be employed but with copious contact jelly to avoid direct pressure on the damaged globe.

Note: In eyes with rupture of the globe, primary closure is required immediately. Vitreoretinal intervention at 2 weeks may be performed, if necessary.

VISUAL OUTCOME

Studies have reported 40% with vision of no light perception (NLP).[33–35] In addition, there may be a cosmetic morbidity with a high risk of phthisis bulbi, occurring in two-thirds of the patients in one study.[35] These eyes often need silicone oil insertion to hold the retina in place (Figure 8.9).

PENETRATING INJURY

CLINICAL PRESENTATION

Sharp instruments may penetrate the sclera in, for example, not only assault with glass bottles or knifes, but also other situations such as working with a screwdriver or other tool usually being used to loosen objects and being drawn back into the eye or even eating utensils.[36] Projectiles such as pellets from air guns cause severe injury with the pellets often stopping at the orbital apex where additional damage is suffered by the optic nerve.[37–39] The tissues damaged depend on the site of entry, depth of penetration and the size of the object. As a result, any intraocular structure may be disrupted. Incarceration sites are problematic when the site of entry involves the posterior sclera, resulting in later retinal detachment as scar tissue contracts pulling in the retina and choroid in a similar mechanism to rupture. There is a high risk of the development of phthisis bulbi.

The injury can cause GRTs.[40]

Introduction of materials such as cilia[41,42] or fly larvae into the eye[43] risks endophthalmitis.

ENDOPHTHALMITIS

Endophthalmitis may complicate any penetrating injury and is seen in approximately 7%,[44] with 20% having virulent organisms.[45] Species of streptococcus, staphylococcus and bacillus are common in adults, with streptococcus most common in children.[46–48] *Bacillus cereus* is highly virulent and a very rare presentation of endophthalmitis without trauma.[49,50] In trauma, unusual organisms not usually seen in infection of the eye can be detected.[51] Prophylactic intravitreal antibiotics have been reported to reduce endophthalmitis rates from 18% to 6% in a study from India.[52]

RETINAL DETACHMENT

Many types of retinal break are found in these traumatised eyes; they may develop at the time of impact or penetration or subsequently from incarceration of the retina.

Penetrating trauma can tear the retina at the site of injury or may produce an incarceration of vitreous, retina and choroid. The latter progressively contracts, shortening the vitreous and retina.

VISUAL OUTCOME

These types of injury are associated with a poor visual outcome with 20/200 or worse vision in 78%, only 60% achieving a flat retina. Phthisis bulbi occurs in 28%.[53] Poor starting vision, the presence of a relative afferent pupillary defect and a large or posterior wound are reported to result in poorer prognosis.[54,55]

TRAUMA SCORES

There are two models for the prediction of visual outcome in open globe injury, the ocular trauma score (OTS) and the classification and regression tree[56,57]; both have been found to be predictive of outcome (Tables 8.3 through 8.5).[58]

Table 8.3 Ocular trauma score

Initial visual acuity	Raw points
1. Initial visual acuity	NLP = 60
	LP to HM = 70
	1/200–19/200 = 80
	20/200–20/50 = 90
	≥20/40 = 100
2. Globe rupture	−23
3. Endophthalmitis	−17
4. Perforating injury	−14
5. Retinal detachment	−11
6. Afferent pupillary defect	−10
Raw score = sum of raw points	

Source: *Ophthalmol Clin North Am*, 15, Kuhn, F. et al., The Ocular Trauma Score (OTS), 163–5, vi, Copyright (2002), with permission from Elsevier.
Note: Calculate the score for the traumatised eye.
Abbreviations: HM, hand motions; LP, light perception; NLP, no light perception.

Table 8.4 Alternative ocular trauma score

Raw sum score	OTS score	NLP (%)	LP/HM (%)	1/200–19/200 (%)	20/2000–20/50 (%)	≥20/40 (%)
0–44	1	73	17	7	2	1
45–65	2	28	26	18	13	15
66–80	3	2	11	15	28	44
81–91	4	1	2	2	21	74
92–100	5	0	1	2	5	92

Note: Probability of achieving a visual acuity depending on the score attained.
Abbreviations: HM, hand motions; LP, light perception; NLP, no light perception.

Table 8.5 Penetrating

Condition	Characteristic	Referral	Why?
Trauma	Penetrating	Emergency	Needs primary repair and antibiotics

INTRAOCULAR FOREIGN BODIES

CLINICAL PRESENTATION

IOFBs are typically caused by striking metal on metal such as hitting a hammer on a chisel, but IOFBs have been described from a wide variety of presentations, such as glass from car windscreens,[10] plastic from fireworks and strimmers,[59] organic material in rural settings, shot gun pellets,[60,61] graphite pencil lead[62] and fragments from lawn mower blades.[63] The diagnosis of ocular retention of a small foreign body (FB) depends on careful attention to the history of the injury. On examination, look for evidence of ocular penetration, such as a small entry site in the anterior sclera or signs of vitreous disturbance such as VH. Posterior segment damage after FB penetration not only is at the site of impaction but may also be found at a site of a ricochet. Local tissue whitening may be visible.

If the retina is damaged, RRD is reported in 25%.[64] However, IOFBs may sit in the vitreous cavity or on the surface of the retina without causing retinal tear. Fibrosis may occur either locally or at the impact site. Visual loss depends on the site of impaction (macular, papillary or peripheral), on the production of opacities in the media (cataract or VH) or on the development of retinal detachment (Figures 8.10 through 8.12).

DIAGNOSTIC IMAGING

1. CT scanning, with thin sections, is the investigation of choice, especially if the IOFB cannot be seen on fundoscopy.
2. Plain X-ray can be used for screening for a suspected FB.
3. Ultrasound examination may be valuable for detecting non-radiolucent foreign bodies, but may not detect small metallic foreign bodies, especially if they are embedded in the ocular tissues. Foreign bodies can give rise to high-amplitude echoes provided they are appropriately orientated to the sound beam; the main value of ultrasound is in determining the vitreoretinal complications of FB impaction such as haemorrhage and retinal detachment.

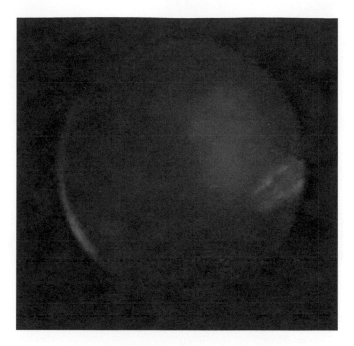

Figure 8.10 IOFB on the retina.

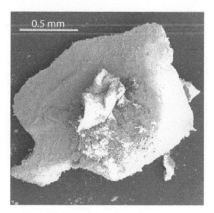

Figure 8.11 Scanning electron microscopy of a metallic IOFB.

A ferromagnetic IOFB is an absolute contraindication to magnetic resonance imaging scanning in case the particle rotates or moves in the magnetic field.

IOFB MATERIALS

The surgical removal of the FB is indicated because of the risk of generalised posterior segment complications such as severe vitritis and endophthalmitis (from bacterial or toxic chemical penetration along with the FB or acute chalcosis). Copper-containing IOFBs cause chalcosis, which can be rapidly damaging to the eye if the copper content of the IOFB is 85% or more.[65] Siderosis results from the chemical destruction and cellular absorption of retained ferrous material.

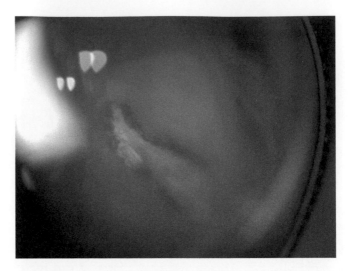

Figure 8.12 Scar in the retina from the impact site of an IOFB.

Table 8.6 Penetrating with IOFB

Condition	Characteristic	Referral	Why?
Trauma	Penetrating with IOFB	Emergency	Needs antibiotics then IOFB removal

The siderosis is slow in onset and can minimally affect vision, giving a tonic pupil, greenish tinge to the iris and late onset cataract formation.[66,67] Retinal damage appears over weeks; some patients may have only mild loss of vision after years. Electroretinography demonstrates reduction in retinal function with reduced amplitudes. The IOFB may dissolve over years, making it undetectable on ophthalmoscopy or CT scan.

Endophthalmitis occurs in 5–7% of cases.[68,69]

Emergency referral is required for the insertion of intravitreal antibiotics urgently. Often, the globe laceration needs to be repaired at presentation followed by simultaneous or later surgery for the removal of the IOFB.

VISUAL OUTCOME

IOFBs have a less severe outcome than other presentations of severe ocular trauma, 27% deteriorating to 20/200 or worse vision and 50% achieving 20/40 vision or better.[70] The visual outcome is worse when retinal detachment, a large IOFB or additional anterior segment injury is present (Table 8.6).[69]

PERFORATING INJURY

Perforating injury occurs when a projectile enters the eye anteriorly and exits posteriorly. It has a very high retinal detachment rate. Only one third achieve moderate vision.[54,71]

This may occur from the following:

1. FB entering and exiting the eye and remaining in the orbit, e.g. shot gun pellet and air rifle pellet. Repair of the eye is required, but the FB can be left in the orbit.

2. IOFB entering the eye perforating the scleral posteriorly but remaining in situ in the posterior sclera, e.g. fragment of metal from hammer and chisel.
3. Injury with a long sharp instrument entering the eye deep enough to injure the posterior sclera.

Sometimes, the exit wound at the posterior of the eye is found unexpectedly during surgery. Often, there is incarceration of tissue, which self-seals the exit wound. There is a high risk of traction from the incarceration site.

SYMPATHETIC OPHTHALMIA

This is a panuveitis of both the affected and fellow eye stimulated by the exposure of intraocular antigens to the immune system and is seen in severe open globe trauma and after repeated posterior segment surgery. Look for deep white spots in the retina (Dalen Fuchs nodules). The risk after trauma in the modern setting appears to be rare (0.1–0.3%)[72–74] and may be more common after posterior segment surgery, i.e. PPV, than after trauma.[75] The improved control of the condition with immune suppression, better visual outcome and a reduction in the number of cases have caused a shift away from primary enucleation (removal of the eye at presentation) as a method to prevent the uveitis.

PROLIFERATIVE VITREORETINOPATHY

The incidence of PVR with the different presentation patterns is shown in Table 8.7,[76] with VH as a strong predictor of its development. PVR reduces the ability to reattach the retina and is associated with poorer anatomical and visual outcomes.

PHTHISIS BULBI

In severely damaged eyes, the damage to the ciliary body causes hypotony. Hypotony may cause tenderness of the eye, and pseudoptosis can occur from shrinkage of the globe size. If cyclitic membranes are present, these can be dissected and segmented in an attempt to regain some function of the ciliary body.[77,78] Ultimately, phthisis bulbi occurs where the eye is shrunken. Cosmetically, this is a poor outcome. Evisceration or enucleation (and its attendant orbital fat atrophy) is very rarely required.

Band keratopathy in damaged eyes is common. This may cause intermittent epithelial breakdown causing pain, usually a severe sudden onset pain lasting a few hours at a time. It can be treated with excimer laser ablation (Figure 8.13).

Table 8.7 PVR and trauma

	Frequency of PVR (%)	Median duration until PVR develops (months)
Perforation	43	1.3
Rupture	21	2.1
Penetration	15	3.2
IOFB	11	3.1
Contusion	1	5.7

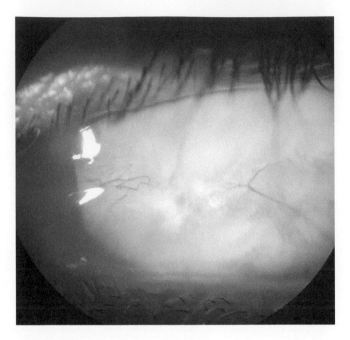

Figure 8.13 Eye in which hypotony has led to phthisis bulbi.

REFERRAL

In most cases, referral is as an emergency for assessment and surgical intervention.

1. Contusion injury should be treated conservatively with complications such as VH and retinal detachment operated upon as indicated.
   a. Retinal dialysis, the most common cause of a late onset retinal detachment, is easily treated by cryotherapy and explant.
   b. GRTs require vitrectomy and endotamponade often with silicone oil insertion.
   c. If a ragged tear of the retina occurs in traumatised retina, often these can be observed and treated only if extension to a retinal detachment occurs.
   d. Macular holes can spontaneously close or be closed by vitrectomy and gas.[79]
2. Rupture requires immediate identification and repair by surgical exploration of the globe at presentation. Thereafter, the eye can be operated upon at 1–2 weeks for complications such as VH or retinal detachment. If the rupture has involved the choroid and retina, often, surgery will be required to relieve traction on the retina by surgical relieving retinectomy, perhaps with choroidectomy in addition.
3. For IOFB, the entry wound should be closed in the first instance with intravitreal antibiotics inserted. Most can be removed on the next day using vitrectomy.
4. Penetrating injury requires immediate repair and intravitreal antibiotics because of a risk of bacterial endophthalmitis. If the injury has involved the choroid and retina, often, surgery will be required to relieve traction on the retina by relieving retinectomy in a similar fashion to rupture.

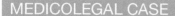

MEDICOLEGAL CASE

CASE 1

A patient is hit in the eye by a sharp piece of metal while using a motorised metal cutter. There is a laceration of the cornea, cataract formation and VH. The patient undergoes a surgical repair of the cornea with nylon sutures, cataract extraction and vitrectomy. The patient is reviewed, and some of the nylon sutures are removed. He is discharged from review.

A few years later, he experiences pain in the eye and face. He is referred to pain management and treated with analgesia, including opiates. Some months later, he is referred back to ophthalmology and a persistent nylon suture is removed and the pain is relieved.

The primary care team in the latter stages did not consider the previous surgery and the possibility that this might be contributing to the pain that this patient was experiencing. There were errors from the ophthalmological team, who should have warned the patient of the possibility of loosening of any residual nylon sutures or provided review of the patient in case of suture problems.

CASE 2

A patient is hit in the eye by a paintball when he lifts his goggles during a paintball party. He is seen with severe injury to the eye with periorbital haemorrhage and severe hyphaema and VH. The patient attends on Saturday evening. The eye is examined by an on-call ophthalmology team, and the patient is booked for review in 1 week. The eye is treated with topical steroids.

After 4 weeks, the patient is referred to the vitreoretinal team for management of a non-clearing VH. On examination, a scleral rupture is suspected from the mode of injury and the severity of the ocular injury. Ultrasound suggests total retinal detachment with PVR. The patient proceeds to surgical exploration of the eye. The lens of the eye is found encapsulated in fibrous tissue under the superior rectus, and a large scleral rupture is detected. This is repaired with suturing. A vitrectomy is performed. Total retinal detachment is detected and is operated upon with silicone oil insertion but with poor visual recovery.

The referral for exploration of the eye was too slow. The initial ophthalmology team did not suspect rupture of the globe.

The timing of surgical intervention in these cases is crucial for maximising outcome, and it was compromised in this case.

REFERENCES

1. Parver, L. M., Dannenberg, A. L., Blacklow, B. et al. Characteristics and causes of penetrating eye injuries reported to the National Eye Trauma System Registry, 1985–91. *Public Health Rep* 1993;108(5):625–32.
2. Tielsch, J. M., Parver, L. and Shankar, B. Time trends in the incidence of hospitalized ocular trauma. *Arch Ophthalmol* 1989;107(4):519–23.
3. Tielsch, J. M. and Parver, L. M. Determinants of hospital charges and length of stay for ocular trauma. *Ophthalmology* 1990;97(2):231–7.

4. Canavan, Y. M., O'Flaherty, M. J., Archer, D. B. and Elwood, J. H. A 10-year survey of eye injuries in Northern Ireland, 1967–76. *Br J Ophthalmol* 1980;64(8):618–25.

5. Schein, O. D., Hibberd, P. L., Shingleton, B. J. et al. The spectrum and burden of ocular injury. *Ophthalmology* 1988;95(3):300–5.

6. Liggett, P. E., Pince, K. J., Barlow, W. et al. Ocular trauma in an urban population. Review of 1132 cases. *Ophthalmology* 1990;97(5):581–4.

7. Khatry, S. K., Lewis, A. E., Schein, O. D. et al. The epidemiology of ocular trauma in rural Nepal. *Br J Ophthalmol* 2004;88(4):456–60.

8. Appiah, A. P. The nature, causes, and visual outcome of ocular trauma requiring posterior segment surgery at a county hospital. *Ann Ophthalmol* 1991;23(11):430–3.

9. Ahmadieh, H., Soheilian, M., Sajjadi, H. et al. Vitrectomy in ocular trauma: Factors influencing final visual outcome. *Retina* 1993;13(2):107–13.

10. Ghoraba, H. Posterior segment glass intraocular foreign bodies following car accident or explosion. *Graefes Arch Clin Exp Ophthalmol* 2002;240(7):524–8.

11. Alfaro, D. V., Chaudhry, N. A., Walonker, A. F. et al. Penetrating eye injuries in young children. *Retina* 1994;14(3):201–5.

12. May, D. R., Kuhn, F. P., Morris, R. E. et al. The epidemiology of serious eye injuries from the United States Eye Injury Registry. *Graefes Arch Clin Exp Ophthalmol* 2000;238(2):153–7.

13. Kuhn, F., Morris, R., Witherspoon, C. D. et al. A standardized classification of ocular trauma. *Ophthalmology* 1996;103(2):240–3.

14. Han, D. P. Retinal detachment caused by air bag injury. *Arch Ophthalmol* 1993;111(10):1317–8.

15. Pieramici, D. J. and Kuhn, F. Frontal air bags and eye injury patterns in automobile crashes. *Arch Ophthalmol* 2003;121(12):1807–8.

16. Pearlman, J. A., Au Eong, K. G., Kuhn, F. and Pieramici, D. J. Airbags and eye injuries: Epidemiology, spectrum of injury, and analysis of risk factors. *Surv Ophthalmol* 2001;46(3):234–42.

17. Mason, J. O. III, Feist, R. M. and White, M. F. Jr. Ocular trauma from paintball-pellet war games. *South Med J* 2002;95(2):218–22.

18. Cooney, M. J. and Pieramici, D. J. Eye injuries caused by bungee cords. *Ophthalmology* 1997;104(10):1644–7.

19. Peyman, G. A., Raichand, M., Goldberg, M. F. and Brown, S. Vitrectomy in the management of intraocular foreign bodies and their complications. *Br J Ophthalmol* 1980;64(7):476–82.

20. Coleman, D. J. Early vitrectomy in the management of the severely traumatized eye. *Am J Ophthalmol* 1982;93(5):543–51.

21. Conway, B. P. and Michels, R. G. Vitrectomy techniques in the management of selected penetrating ocular injuries. *Ophthalmology* 1978;85(6):560–83.

22. Ryan, S. J. Results of pars plana vitrectomy in penetrating ocular trauma. *Int Ophthalmol* 1978;1(1):5–8.

23. Mody, K. V., Blach, R. K., Leaver, P. K. and McLeod, D. Closed vitrectomy after trauma. *Trans Ophthalmol Soc UK* 1978;98(1):55–8.

24. Mandelcorn, M. S. Results after vitrectomy in trauma. *Can J Ophthalmol* 1977;12(1):34–7.

25. Hutton, W. L., Snyder, W. B. and Vaiser, A. Vitrectomy in the treatment of ocular perforating injuries. *Am J Ophthalmol* 1976;81(6):733–9.

26. Pieramici, D. J., MacCumber, M. W., Humayun, M. U. et al. Open-globe injury: Update on types of injuries and visual results. *Ophthalmology* 1996;103(11):1798–803.

27. Qiang Kwong, T., Shunmugam, M. and Williamson, T. H. Characteristics of rheg-matogenous retinal detachments secondary to retinal dialyses. *Can J Ophthalmol* 2014;49(2):196–9.

28. Alappatt, J. J. and Hutchins, R. K. Retinal detachments due to traumatic tears in the pars plana ciliaris. *Retina* 1998;18(6):506–9.

29. Martin, D. F., Awh, C. C., McCuen, B. W. et al. Treatment and pathogenesis of traumatic chorioretinal rupture (sclopetaria). *Am J Ophthalmol* 1994;117(2):190–200.

30. Russell, S. R., Olsen, K. R. and Folk, J. C. Predictors of scleral rupture and the role of vitrectomy in severe blunt ocular trauma. *Am J Ophthalmol* 1988;105(3):253–7.

31. Joseph, D. P., Pieramici, D. J. and Beauchamp, N. J. Jr. Computed tomography in the diagnosis and prognosis of open-globe injuries. *Ophthalmology* 2000;107(10):1899–906.

32. Winthrop, S. R., Cleary, P. E., Minckler, D. S. and Ryan, S. J. Penetrating eye injuries: A histopathological review. *Br J Ophthalmol* 1980;64(11):809–17.

33. Morris, R. E., Witherspoon, C. D., Helms, H. A. Jr. et al. Eye Injury Registry of Alabama (preliminary report): Demographics and prognosis of severe eye injury. *South Med J* 1987;80(7):810–6.

34. Soheilian, M., Peyman, G. A., Wafapoor, H. et al. Surgical management of trau-matic retinal detachment with perfluorocarbon liquid: The Vitreon Study Group. *Int Ophthalmol* 1996;20(5):241–9.

35. Liggett, P. E., Gauderman, W. J., Moreira, C. M. et al. Pars plana vitrectomy for acute retinal detachment in penetrating ocular injuries. *Arch Ophthalmol* 1990;108(12):1724–8.

36. Feist, R. M., Lim, J. I., Joondeph, B. C. et al. Penetrating ocular injury from contaminated eating utensils. *Arch Ophthalmol* 1991;109(1):63–6.

37. Pulido, J. S., Gupta, S., Folk, J. C. and Ossoiny, K. C. Perforating BB gun injuries of the globe. *Ophthalmic Surg Lasers* 1997;28(8):625–32.

38. Enger, C., Schein, O. D. and Tielsch, J. M. Risk factors for ocular injuries caused by air guns. *Arch Ophthalmol* 1996;114(4):469–74.

39. Schein, O. D., Enger, C. and Tielsch, J. M. The context and consequences of ocular inju-ries from air guns. *Am J Ophthalmol* 1994;117(4):501–6.

40. Aylward, G. W., Cooling, R. J. and Leaver, P. K. Trauma-induced retinal detachment associated with giant retinal tears. *Retina* 1993;13(2):136–41.

41. Gupta, A. K., Ghosh, B., Mazumdar, S. and Gupta, A. An unusual intraocular foreign body. *Acta Ophthalmol Scand* 1996;74(2):200–1.

42. Fortuin, M. E. and Blanksma, L. J. An unusual complication of perforating wounds of the eye. *Doc Ophthalmol* 1986;61(3–4):197–203.

43. Gozum, N., Kir, N. and Ovali, T. Internal ophthalmomyiasis presenting as endo-phthalmitis associated with an intraocular foreign body. *Ophthalmic Surg Las Im* 2003;34(6):472–4.

44. Essex, R. W., Yi, Q., Charles, P. G. and Allen, P. J. Post-traumatic endophthalmitis. *Ophthalmology* 2004;111(11):2015–22.

45. Lieb, D. F., Scott, I. U., Flynn, H. W. Jr. et al. Open globe injuries with positive intra-ocular cultures: Factors influencing final visual acuity outcomes. *Ophthalmology* 2003;110(8):1560–6.

46. Miller, J. J., Scott, I. U., Flynn, H. W. Jr. et al. Endophthalmitis caused by *Bacillus* species. *Am J Ophthalmol* 2008;145(5):883–8.

47. Alfaro, D. V., Roth, D. and Liggett, P. E. Posttraumatic endophthalmitis: Causative organisms, treatment, and prevention. *Retina* 1994;14(3):206–11.

48. Alfaro, D. V., Roth, D. B., Laughlin, R. M. et al. Paediatric post-traumatic endophthalmitis. *Br J Ophthalmol* 1995;79(10):888–91.

49. Reynolds, D. S. and Flynn, H. W. Jr. Endophthalmitis after penetrating ocular trauma. *Curr Opin Ophthalmol* 1997;8(3):32–8.

50. Foster, R. E., Martinez, J. A., Murray, T. G. et al. Useful visual outcomes after treatment of *Bacillus cereus* endophthalmitis. *Ophthalmology* 1996;103(3):390–7.

51. Essex, R. W., Charles, P. G. and Allen, P. J. Three cases of post-traumatic endophthalmitis caused by unusual bacteria. *Clin Experiment Ophthalmol* 2004;32(4):445–7.

52. Narang, S., Gupta, V., Gupta, A. et al. Role of prophylactic intravitreal antibiotics in open globe injuries. *Indian J Ophthalmol* 2003;51(1):39–44.

53. Meredith, T. A. and Gordon, P. A. Pars plana vitrectomy for severe penetrating injury with posterior segment involvement. *Am J Ophthalmol* 1987;103(4):549–54.

54. Pieramici, D. J., Eong, K. G., Sternberg, P. Jr. and Marsh, M. J. The prognostic significance of a system for classifying mechanical injuries of the eye (globe) in open-globe injuries. *J Trauma* 2003;54(4):750–4.

55. Esmaeli, B., Elner, S. G., Schork, M. A. and Elner, V. M. Visual outcome and ocular survival after penetrating trauma: A clinicopathologic study. *Ophthalmology* 1995;102(3):393–400.

56. Kuhn, F., Maisiak, R., Mann, L. et al. The Ocular Trauma Score (OTS). *Ophthalmol Clin North Am* 2002;15(2):163–5, vi.

57. Schmidt, G. W., Broman, A. T., Hindman, H. B. and Grant, M. P. Vision survival after open globe injury predicted by classification and regression tree analysis. *Ophthalmology* 2008;115(1):202–9.

58. Man, C. Y. and Steel, D. Visual outcome after open globe injury: A comparison of two prognostic models – The Ocular Trauma Score and the Classification and Regression Tree. *Eye (Lond)* 2010;24(1):84–9.

59. Lambert, H. M. and Sipperley, J. O. Intraocular foreign body from a nylon line grass trimmer. *Ann Ophthalmol* 1983;15(10):936–7.

60. Alfaro, D. V., Tran, V. T., Runyan, T. et al. Vitrectomy for perforating eye injuries from shotgun pellets. *Am J Ophthalmol* 1992;114(1):81–5.

61. Morris, R. E., Witherspoon, C. D., Feist, R. M. et al. Bilateral ocular shotgun injury. *Am J Ophthalmol* 1987;103(5):695–700.

62. Hamanaka, N., Ikeda, T., Inokuchi, N. et al. A case of an intraocular foreign body due to graphite pencil lead complicated by endophthalmitis. *Ophthalmic Surg Lasers* 1999;30(3):229–31.

63. John, G., Witherspoon, C. D., Feist, R. M. and Morris, R. Ocular lawnmower injuries. *Ophthalmology* 1988;95(10):1367–70.

64. Ahmadieh, H., Sajjadi, H., Azarmina, M. et al. Surgical management of intraretinal foreign bodies. *Retina* 1994;14(5):397–403.

65. Billi, B., Lesnoni, G., Scassa, C. et al. Copper intraocular foreign body: Diagnosis and treatment. *Eur J Ophthalmol* 1995;5(4):235–9.

66. Weiss, M. J., Hofeldt, A. J., Behrens, M. and Fisher, K. Ocular siderosis: Diagnosis and management. *Retina* 1997;17(2):105–8.

67. Sneed, S. R. and Weingeist, T. A. Management of siderosis bulbi due to a retained iron-containing intraocular foreign body. *Ophthalmology* 1990;97(3):375–9.

68. Thompson, J. T., Parver, L. M., Enger, C. L. et al. Infectious endophthalmitis after penetrating injuries with retained intraocular foreign bodies: National Eye Trauma System. *Ophthalmology* 1993;100(10):1468–74.

69. Jonas, J. B., Knorr, H. L. and Budde, W. M. Prognostic factors in ocular injuries caused by intraocular or retrobulbar foreign bodies. *Ophthalmology* 2000;107(5):823–8.

70. Wani, V. B., Al Ajmi, M., Thalib, L. et al. Vitrectomy for posterior segment intraocular foreign bodies: Visual results and prognostic factors. *Retina* 2003;23(5):654–60.

71. Ramsay, R. C., Cantrill, H. L. and Knobloch, W. H. Vitrectomy for double penetrating ocular injuries. *Am J Ophthalmol* 1985;100(4):586–9.

72. Allen, J. C. Sympathetic ophthalmia, a disappearing disease. *JAMA* 1969;209(7):1090.

73. Kraus-Mackiw, E. Prevention of sympathetic ophthalmia: State of the art 1989. *Int Ophthalmol* 1990;14(5–6):391–4.

74. Liddy, L. and Stuart, J. Sympathetic ophthalmia in Canada. *Can J Ophthalmol* 1972;7(2):157–9.

75. Kilmartin, D. J., Dick, A. D. and Forrester, J. V. Prospective surveillance of sympathetic ophthalmia in the UK and Republic of Ireland. *Br J Ophthalmol* 2000;84(3):259–63.

76. Cardillo, J. A., Stout, J. T., LaBree, L. et al. Post-traumatic proliferative vitreoretinopathy. The epidemiologic profile, onset, risk factors, and visual outcome. *Ophthalmology* 1997;104(7):1166–73.

77. Essex, R. W., Tufail, A., Bunce, C. and Aylward, G. W. Two-year results of surgical removal of choroidal neovascular membranes related to non-age-related macular degeneration. *Br J Ophthalmol* 2007;91(5):649–54.

78. Banaee, T., Ahmadieh, H., Abrishami, M. and Moosavi, M. Removal of traumatic cyclitic membranes: Surgical technique and results. *Graefes Arch Clin Exp Ophthalmol* 2007;245(3):443–7.

79. Kuhn, F., Morris, R., Mester, V. and Witherspoon C. D. Internal limiting membrane removal for traumatic macular holes. *Ophthalmic Surg Lasers* 2001;32(4):308–15.

Complications of anterior segment surgery

INTRODUCTION

Cataract surgery is performed by phacoemulsification with a small incision and a sutureless wound. This is the most common operation on the eye, and therefore, you may encounter patients with complications from this procedure. In general, it is a safe operation with a high rate of success, approximately 95%. However, there remains a small complication rate of approximately 2%.

Some of these are serious complications and will often involve the vitreoretinal surgeon in remedying the situation.

DROPPED NUCLEUS

CLINICAL FEATURES

The dropped nucleus incidence is 0.09–0.8%.[1–4]

The phrase 'dropped nucleus' has been used to describe the dislocation of the nucleus (or part of the nucleus) of a cataract into the vitreous cavity during phacoemulsification surgery. Dropped nucleus may happen to any case, but certain cases are more at risk:

- Trauma
- Pseudoexfoliation
- Hard nuclei
- Inexperienced surgeon[1]

The positive pressure applied by the infusion fluid during phacoemulsification means that a tear in the posterior capsule of the lens can enlarge and result in the dislocation of the lens nucleus into the vitreous cavity. The nucleus is denser than the vitreous and therefore drops to the posterior pole (Figures 9.1 through 9.3).

The lens material causes the following:

- *Uveitis (56%):* This is seen early. The nuclear fragment can persist for months creating a chronic uveitis, which may persist after remedial surgery.[5]

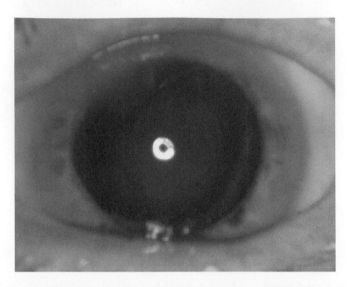

Figure 9.1 Anterior segment of an eye after a recent complicated cataract operation. There is some soft lens material, and the capsule is torn. No lens implant has been inserted.

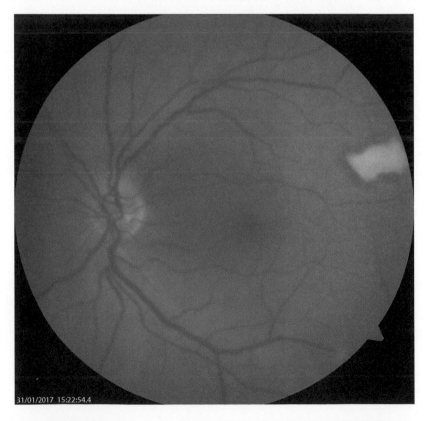

Figure 9.2 Fragment of the nucleus in the vitreous after a complicated cataract operation.

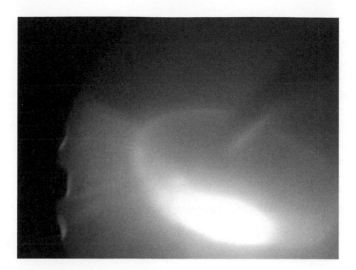

Figure 9.3 Nucleus of a cataract has dropped into the posterior segment and is being removed during vitrectomy.

- *Glaucoma (52%):* A severe rise in IOP must be controlled by topical medication but requires removal of the nucleus to cure. Again, if the nucleus remains in the eye for a prolonged period, the glaucoma may not reverse after lens removal.
- *Retinal detachment:* The disruption to the vitreous may produce retinal detachment by retinal tear formation, seen in 4–8% of patients.[6,7] There is an increased risk of RRD approximately 4% at presentation, but even after the removal of the nucleus, RRD can occur in 4%.[8] Post-operative RRD is reported earlier in these patients (mean: 4 months) than after routine cataract extraction (mean: 16 months).[9]

PPV and the removal of the nucleus are required within 1 or 2 weeks to avoid glaucomatous damage or chronic uveitis or cystoid macular oedema (CMO).[10] Rarely, dropped nucleus can present with endophthalmitis[11] with the risk of endophthalmitis doubled over other surgery.[12]

SUCCESS RATES

Visual outcome is approximately a 60% chance of 20/40 vision or better, which is approximately 20% less than after routine cataract extraction (Table 9.1).[8,13,14]

Table 9.1 Referral for dropped nucleus

Condition	Characteristics	Referral	Why?
Dropped nucleus	All	1 week	Needs surgery promptly because of uveitis, glaucoma and occasionally retinal detachment
Complicated cataract operation		Routine referral for assessment	Risk of RRD

INTRAOCULAR LENS DISLOCATIONS

CLINICAL PRESENTATION

A prosthetic intraocular lens (IOL) implant can also dislocate into the posterior segment, spontaneously, after minor trauma from predisposing conditions, such as pseudoexfoliation or high myopia, or because of complications from the cataract surgery. Silicone plate IOLs were particularly prone to this after yttrium aluminium garnet (YAG) capsulotomy (typically at 2 months after the laser procedure).[15,16] This requires not only remedial surgery to remove the IOL but also specialised techniques to insert and fixate a new IOL. The eye is surprisingly tolerant to the dislocated IOL in the posterior segment, but there is a worry about trauma to the surface of the retina and a risk of retinal detachment. Therefore, prompt referral for assessment is prudent (Figures 9.4 and 9.5) (Table 9.2).

POST-OPERATIVE ENDOPHTHALMITIS

CLINICAL FEATURES

The incidence of endophthalmitis in cataract surgery is 0.028–0.14%.[17–19]

If a patient experiences severe pain in the first week after cataract surgery (3–5 days), the eye must be examined as quickly as possible for endophthalmitis. The sooner that the eye receives intraocular antibiotics, the greater the chance of recovery, so immediate referral is required. The patient often experiences a drop in vision usually accompanied by an aching pain in the eye. The eye is inflamed with signs of anterior uveitis (cells and flare), followed by the formation of a hypopyon (a layer of white cells in the inferior anterior chamber). Fibrin may be deposited on the lens implant and the iris blood vessels engorged. A view of the retina may not be possible because of the infiltration of the vitreous with white cells, but a red reflex may be visible. If the retina can be observed, sheathing of the blood vessels and retinal haemorrhaging indicate vasculitis and a poorer prognosis for visual recovery (Figures 9.6 and 9.7).

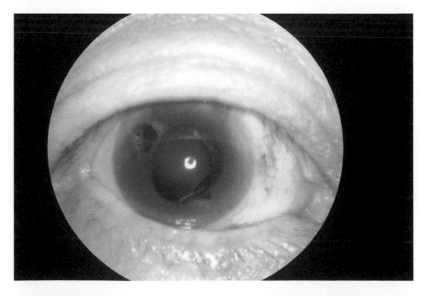

Figure 9.4 Sulcus-placed IOL is subluxated after complicated cataract surgery.

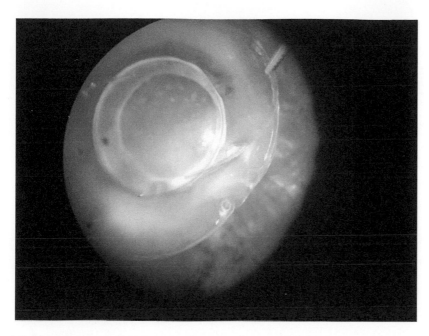

Figure 9.5 Dislocated IOL in the vitreous cavity. The zonules have broken, and the capsule and IOL dropped into the posterior segment.

Table 9.2 Dislocated IOL

Condition	Characteristics	Referral	Why?
Dislocated IOL	All	Prompt referral within a week or two	Risk of RRD

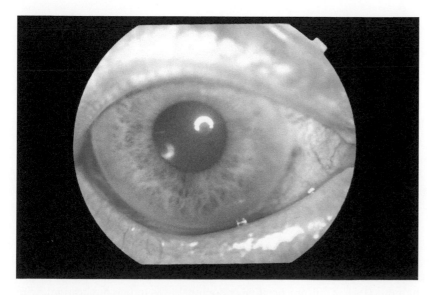

Figure 9.6 Early hypopyon in a post-opertive endophthalmitis.

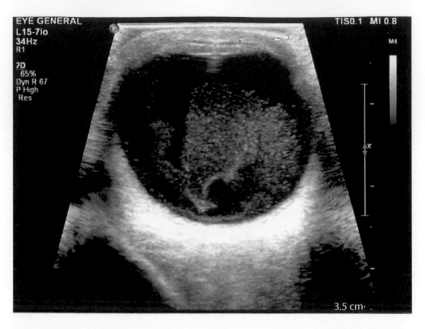

Figure 9.7 Ultrasound of an eye with endophthalmitis after an intravitreal steroid inection. The vitreous is opacified by white blood cells but remains attached.

Hypopyon and pain are not always present.[20]

The priority in the management of the patient is to inject intravitreal antibiotics as soon as possible.

Blebitis (infection of the drainage bleb) in patients with trabeculectomy may also lead to late endophthalmitis months or years after the surgery.

The risk of retinal detachment is 8.3% in post-operative endophthalmitis.[21]

INFECTIVE ORGANISMS

Fifty-six to 69% of samples are culture positive.[18,22]

- Virulent bacteria
  - *Staphylococcus aureus*
  - *Streptococcus pyogenes*
  - *Hemophilus influenzae*[23]
  - Coliforms
  - *Pseudomonas aeruginosa*[24]
  - Klebsiella[25]
- Less virulent bacteria
  - *Staphylococcus epidermidis* (coagulase-negative staphylococci)
  - *Proprionibacterium acnes*[26]

The less virulent organisms have a much better visual prognosis. Coagulase-negative staphylococci are the commonest pathogens and may be introduced from the patient's eyelids or conjunctiva.[27] Methicillin-resistant *S. aureus* has been implicated in post-operative endophthalmitis (18% of culture-positive endophthalmitis in one publication), with *in vitro* sensitivity to gentamycin and vancomycin.[28] Very occasionally, fungal post-operative infections are seen.[29]

The frequencies of isolation of organisms in positive biopsies (94% are Gram positive)[22] are as follows:

- Coagulase-negative staphylococci: 70%
- *S. aureus*: 10%
- Streptococci: 9%
- Gram-negative bacteria: 6%
- Enterococci: 2%
- Other Gram-positive bacteria: 3%

S. epidermidis is less common in cases of endophthalmitis related to trabeculectomy.[30]

ANTIBIOTICS

Intravitreal antibiotics are injected and provide a high concentration of drug to treat the infection. For this reason, systemic antibiotics appear to add little to the therapeutic dose.[31] Topical antibiotics will provide additional dosage only to the anterior chamber. Third-generation cephalosporins (useful for Gram-negative organisms) are effective in combination with vancomycin (for Gram-positive organisms) and should remain in the eye for a week at therapeutic doses.[32,33] Eleven per cent of Gram-negative organisms[22] have been described as resistant to cephalosporins, however.

Aminoglycosides (gentamicin and amikacin) have been used in the past but are associated with retinal vascular occlusion in some patients, which causes profound irreversible loss of vision.[34–38]

Intravitreal steroid has been used as an adjunctive treatment but is of uncertain worth.[39]

Repeat biopsy may be required in 10% for worsening inflammation, with a positive culture in 42%. Repeat biopsy is often associated with a poor visual outcome.[40]

SUCCESS RATES

There is a 50% chance of moderate vision, one-third chance of achieving 20/40 vision or better[41,42] and 13% chance of no light perception (NLP) (Table 9.3).[18] Those patients with coagulase-negative staphylococci obtain the best results.

Visual results by organism[43] (rates of 20/100 or better) are as follows:

- Coagulase-negative staphylococci: 84%
- Gram negative: 56%
- *S. aureus*: 50%
- Streptococci: 30%
- Enterococci: 14%

Table 9.3 Post-operative endophthalmitis

Condition	Characteristics	Referral	Why
Post-operative endophthalmitis	All	Emergency referral on the same day	The sooner the antibiotics are inserted, the better the outcome

CHRONIC POST-OPERATIVE ENDOPHTHALMITIS

This often masquerades as a panuveitis post-operatively and should be suspected in a pseudo-phakic eye with chronic inflammation. These eyes may have a white capsular plaque, indicating a focus of infection around the IOL. Chronic endophthalmitis is caused by low-virulence bacteria, classically not only *P. acnes* or *S. epidermidis*, but also occasionally other organisms.

The best results are often obtained by PPV and removal of the IOL and capsule, but these have visual consequences. Despite the eradication of the infection, the patient may still require medical therapy for chronic uveitis and CMO.[26]

NEEDLE-STICK INJURY

CLINICAL FEATURES

Needle-stick injury has the following clinical features:

- Incidence: Globe penetration from the local anaesthetic needle in all patients is 0.014%, and in patients with axial length more than 26 mm, it is 0.7%[44] and posterior staphyloma increases to 0.13%.[45]
- Fifty-three per cent of cases of globe perforation are in myopic eyes.[46]
- Fifty-five per cent of cases are in eyes with normal axial lengths.[44]

Although most cataract operations are performed with anaesthetic drops in most circumstances, orbital injections of anaesthesia are sometimes used. The needle may penetrate the eye in retrobulbar, peribulbar and even subtenon injections.[47] Penetration may cause haemorrhage in the choroid, subretinal space or into the vitreous, and tears in the retina can result in retinal detachment (Table 9.4). A vitrectomy to clear out VH and to allow visualisation of the retina may be required. There is a 40% chance of PVR[44,45] if RRD occurs.

The incarceration sites from needle-stick injuries are usually small but may be multiple as the person anaesthetising repeatedly inserts the needle while trying to reach the posterior orbit. If an attempt has been made to inject the local anaesthesia while the needle tip is in the eye, the pressure rise can induce a scleral rupture similar to a blunt trauma.[48,49] The need for vitrectomy depends on the presence of VH or retinal detachment. PPV is required in 40–80%,[50,51] with a 50% chance of 20/40 vision or better.

INTRAOCULAR HAEMORRHAGE

The incidence of choroidal haemorrhage in cataract surgery is 0.04–0.16%.[52,53]

Spontaneous choroidal haemorrhage occurs because of the sudden drop in IOP when the eye is opened during surgery or by distortion of the globe during surgical manoeuvres. Any

Table 9.4 Needle-stick injury

Condition	Characteristics	Referral	Why
Needle-stick injury	All	Prompt referral for assessment	Vitrectomy may be required for complications

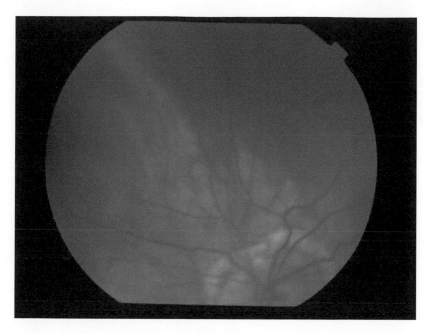

Figure 9.8 Choroidal haemorrhage in a myopic patient.

fragile blood vessels in the choroid may fracture and bleed causing the catastrophic 'expulsive haemorrhage' where the whole of the choroid is elevated by blood. The eyes of patients with high myopia, high IOP, arteriopathy or old age are particularly at risk. The management of the condition is similar to the treatment of choroidal haemorrhage in trauma by waiting for improvement and clearance once haemolysis has commenced (Figure 9.8).

RETINAL DETACHMENT

The following are the 4-year incidence rates of retinal detachment[17]:

- All cataract extractions: 1.17%
- With vitreous loss at the cataract extraction: 4.9%
- Phacoemulsification: 0.4%

(The rates are increased in the white race, the young and those with YAG capsulotomy.)

An increased risk of retinal detachment is associated with a previous cataract extraction operation. Approximately 30% of RRDs are pseudophakic.[54] When the cataract surgery has been complicated by vitreous loss, the vitreous disruption results in a PVD or in further shrinkage of the vitreous and retinal tear formation. However, even uncomplicated cataract surgery seems to induce a risk of retinal detachment. It may be that the loss of the larger volume of the crystalline lens by the lower volume of the IOL implant induces a change in the vitreous, inducing vitreous detachment, which in turn, increases the risk of retinal break formation. The retinal detachment risk appears at a mean of 15 months after the surgery. These patients may experience floaters and flashes but often present late and with their macula detached.

CHRONIC UVEITIS

Some patients may develop chronic uveitis after cataract extraction.
The following are the causes:

- Missed or ignored dropped nuclear fragment
- Piece of nucleus in the angle
- Low-grade endophthalmitis (see Post-operative Endophthalmitis)

POST-OPERATIVE VITREOMACULAR TRACTION

Sudden onset vitreomacular traction can be seen rarely after cataract extraction[55] from the contraction of the vitreous gel in uncomplicated cataract surgery. This presents in the few weeks after surgery and is spontaneously resolved in 50% in a couple of months with separation of the gel, with the remainder requiring PPV.

POST-OPERATIVE CHOROIDAL EFFUSION

Choroidal effusions are smooth elevations of the retina and choroid and have a deep green colour. They are of thicker consistency than RRD. Effusions will complicate hypotony and are more likely to occur with glaucoma drainage procedures. Most will resolve spontaneously, but others will require drainage and PPV (Figure 9.9).

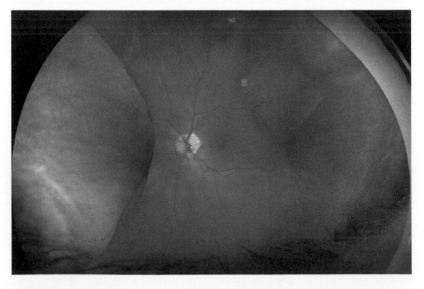

Figure 9.9 Choroidal effusions can be seen in an eye with post-operative hypotony.

MEDICOLEGAL CASE

A patient attends an optometrist, who diagnoses cataracts. She then attends her FP and is referred to ophthalmology routinely for assessment. The patient has bilateral nuclear sclerotic cataracts with pseudoexfoliation. Her visual acuity is significantly impaired to 20/200 vision in each eye. She proceeds to undergo a cataract extraction on the right eye. Recovery is satisfactory, and she is listed for surgery on the left eye. A consent form outlines a number of risks to the surgery. She undergoes phacoemulsification operation on the left eye. There is a posterior capsular tear during surgery, with part of the nucleus dropped into the back of the eye. A decision is taken to wait to see if the dropped nuclear fragment will disperse.

The IOP elevates and is difficult to control. The patient is then referred to the vitreoretinal team after a delay of 1 month. The fragment is removed from the eye by vitrectomy.

In the post-operative period, the IOP is easier to control but the patient requires continued topical medications. Later it is noted that there is asymmetrical cupping of the optic discs, and a visual field test shows constriction of the visual field on the left eye.

The cataract operations were likely to be difficult with the combination of pseudoexfoliation and severe cataract. Therefore, the complication of a dropped nuclear fragment during cataract surgery cannot be criticized. Referral for the vitrectomy, however, was unnecessarily delayed, resulting in raised IOP and some damage to the eye.

It is preferable to have nuclear fragments removed within 1–2 weeks of the cataract operation.

REFERENCES

1. Aasuri, M. K., Kompella, V. B. and Majji, A. B. Risk factors for and management of dropped nucleus during phacoemulsification. *J Cataract Refract Surg* 2001;27(9):1428–32.
2. Kageyama, T., Ayaki, M., Ogasawara, M. et al. Results of vitrectomy performed at the time of phacoemulsification complicated by intravitreal lens fragments. *Br J Ophthalmol* 2001;85(9):1038–40.
3. Mathai, A. and Thomas, R. Incidence and management of posteriorly dislocated nuclear fragments following phacoemulsification. *Indian J Ophthalmol* 1999;47(3):173–6.
4. Stilma, J. S., van der Sluijs, F. A., van Meurs, J. C. and Mertens, D. A. Occurrence of retained lens fragments after phacoemulsification in the Netherlands. *J Cataract Refract Surg* 1997;23(8):1177–82.
5. Gilliland, G. D., Hutton, W. L. and Fuller, D. G. Retained intravitreal lens fragments after cataract surgery. *Ophthalmology* 1992;99(8):1263–7.
6. Ross, W. H. Management of dislocated lens fragments after phacoemulsification surgery. *Can J Ophthalmol* 1996;31(5):234–40.
7. Oruc, S. and Kaplan, H. J. Outcome of vitrectomy for retained lens fragments after phacoemulsification. *Ocul Immunol Inflamm* 2001;9(1):41–7.
8. Hansson, L. J. and Larsson, J. Vitrectomy for retained lens fragments in the vitreous after phacoemulsification. *J Cataract Refract Surg* 2002;28(6):1007–11.
9. Haddad, W. M., Monin, C., Morel, C. et al. Retinal detachment after phacoemulsification: A study of 114 cases. *Am J Ophthalmol* 2002;133(5):630–8.
10. Rossetti, A. and Doro, D. Retained intravitreal lens fragments after phacoemulsification: Complications and visual outcome in vitrectomized and nonvitrectomized eyes. *J Cataract Refract Surg* 2002;28(2):310–5.

11. Irvine, W. D., Flynn, H. W. Jr., Murray, T. G. and Rubsamen, P. E. Retained lens fragments after phacoemulsification manifesting as marked intraocular inflammation with hypopyon. *Am J Ophthalmol* 1992;114(5):610–4.

12. Kim, J. E., Flynn, H. W. Jr., Rubsamen, P. E. et al. Endophthalmitis in patients with retained lens fragments after phacoemulsification. *Ophthalmology* 1996;103(4):575–8.

13. Kim, J. E., Flynn, H. W. Jr., Smiddy, W. E. et al. Retained lens fragments after phacoemulsification. *Ophthalmology* 1994;101(11):1827–32.

14. Smiddy, W. E., Guererro, J. L., Pinto, R. and Feuer, W. Retinal detachment rate after vitrectomy for retained lens material after phacoemulsification. *Am J Ophthalmol* 2003;135(2):183–7.

15. Agustin, A. L. and Miller, K. M. Posterior dislocation of a plate-haptic silicone intraocular lens with large fixation holes. *J Cataract Refract Surg* 2000;26(9):1428–9.

16. Schneiderman, T. E. and Vine, A. K. Retained lens fragment after phacoemulsification. *Ophthalmology* 1995;102(12):1735–6.

17. Javitt, J. C., Vitale, S., Canner, J. K. et al. National outcomes of cataract extraction: Endophthalmitis following inpatient surgery. *Arch Ophthalmol* 1991;109(8):1085–9.

18. Kamalarajah, S., Silvestri, G., Sharma, N. et al. Surveillance of endophthalmitis following cataract surgery in the UK. *Eye* 2004;18(6):580–7.

19. Wykoff, C. C., Parrott, M. B., Flynn, H. W. Jr. et al. Nosocomial acute-onset postoperative endophthalmitis at a university teaching hospital (2002–2009). *Am J Ophthalmol* 2010;150(3):392–8 e2.

20. Wisniewski, S. R., Capone, A., Kelsey, S. F. et al. Characteristics after cataract extraction or secondary lens implantation among patients screened for the Endophthalmitis Vitrectomy Study. *Ophthalmology* 2000;107(7):1274–82.

21. Doft, B. M., Kelsey, S. F. and Wisniewski, S. R. Retinal detachment in the endophthalmitis vitrectomy study. *Arch Ophthalmol* 2000;118(12):1661–5.

22. Han, D. P., Wisniewski, S. R., Wilson, L. A. et al. Spectrum and susceptibilities of microbiologic isolates in the Endophthalmitis Vitrectomy Study. *Am J Ophthalmol* 1996;122(1):1–17.

23. Yoder, D. M., Scott, I. U., Flynn, H. W. Jr. and Miller, D. Endophthalmitis caused by *Haemophilus influenzae*. *Ophthalmology* 2004;111(11):2023–6.

24. Eifrig, C. W., Scott, I. U., Flynn, H. W. Jr. and Miller, D. Endophthalmitis caused by *Pseudomonas aeruginosa*. *Ophthalmology* 2003;110(9):1714–7.

25. Scott, I. U., Matharoo, N., Flynn, H. W. Jr. and Miller, D. Endophthalmitis caused by Klebsiella species. *Am J Ophthalmol* 2004;138(4):662–3.

26. Meisler, D. M. and Mandelbaum, S. Propionibacterium-associated endophthalmitis after extracapsular cataract extraction: Review of reported cases. *Ophthalmology* 1989;96(1):54–61.

27. Bannerman, T. L., Rhoden, D. L., McAllister, S. K. et al. The source of coagulase-negative staphylococci in the Endophthalmitis Vitrectomy Study: A comparison of eyelid and intraocular isolates using pulsed-field gel electrophoresis. *Arch Ophthalmol* 1997;115(3):357–61.

28. Deramo, V. A., Lai, J. C., Winokur, J. et al. Visual outcome and bacterial sensitivity after methicillin-resistant *Staphylococcus aureus*-associated acute endophthalmitis. *Am J Ophthalmol* 2008;145(3):413–7.

29. Narang, S., Gupta, A., Gupta, V. et al. Fungal endophthalmitis following cataract surgery: Clinical presentation, microbiological spectrum, and outcome. *Am J Ophthalmol* 2001;132(5):609–17.

30. Ciulla, T. A., Beck, A. D., Topping, T. M. and Baker, A. S. Blebitis, early endophthalmitis, and late endophthalmitis after glaucoma-filtering surgery. *Ophthalmology* 1997;104(6):986–95.

31. Results of the Endophthalmitis Vitrectomy Study. A randomized trial of immediate vitrectomy and of intravenous antibiotics for the treatment of postoperative bacterial endophthalmitis. Endophthalmitis Vitrectomy Study Group. *Arch Ophthalmol* 1995; 113(12):1479–96.

32. Ferencz, J. R., Assia, E. I., Diamantstein, L. and Rubinstein, E. Vancomycin concentration in the vitreous after intravenous and intravitreal administration for postoperative endophthalmitis. *Arch Ophthalmol* 1999;117(8):1023–7.

33. Gan, I. M., van Dissel, J. T., Beekhuis, W. H. et al. Intravitreal vancomycin and gentamicin concentrations in patients with postoperative endophthalmitis. *Br J Ophthalmol* 2001;85(11):1289–93.

34. Campochiaro, P. A. and Conway, B. P. Aminoglycoside toxicity – A survey of retinal specialists: Implications for ocular use. *Arch Ophthalmol* 1991;109(7):946–50.

35. Waltz, K. and Margo, C. E. Intraocular gentamicin toxicity. *Arch Ophthalmol* 1991;109(7):911.

36. Jackson, T. L. and Williamson, T. H. Amikacin retinal toxicity. *Br J Ophthalmol* 1999;83(10):1199–200.

37. Campochiaro, P. A. and Lim, J. I. Aminoglycoside toxicity in the treatment of endophthalmitis: The Aminoglycoside Toxicity Study Group. *Arch Ophthalmol* 1994;112(1):48–53.

38. Seawright, A. A., Bourke, R. D. and Cooling, R. J. Macula toxicity after intravitreal amikacin. *Aust NZ J Ophthalmol* 1996;24(2):143–6.

39. Shah, G. K., Stein, J. D., Sharma, S. et al. Visual outcomes following the use of intravitreal steroids in the treatment of postoperative endophthalmitis. *Ophthalmology* 2000;107(3):486–9.

40. Doft, B. H., Kelsey, S. F. and Wisniewski, S. R. Additional procedures after the initial vitrectomy or tap-biopsy in the Endophthalmitis Vitrectomy Study. *Ophthalmology* 1998;105(4):707–16.

41. Ng, J. Q., Morlet, N., Pearman, J. W. et al. Management and outcomes of postoperative endophthalmitis since the Endophthalmitis Vitrectomy Study: The Endophthalmitis Population Study of Western Australia (EPSWA)'s Fifth Report. *Ophthalmology* 2005;112:1119–206.

42. Doft, B. H., Kelsey, S. F., Wisniewski, S. et al. Treatment of endophthalmitis after cataract extraction. *Retina* 1994;14(4):297–304.

43. Durand, M. Microbiologic factors and visual outcome in the endophthalmitis vitrectomy study. *Am J Ophthalmol* 1996;122(6):830–46.

44. Duker, J. S., Belmont, J. B., Benson, W. E. et al. Inadvertent globe perforation during retrobulbar and peribulbar anesthesia: Patient characteristics, surgical management, and visual outcome. *Ophthalmology* 1991;98(4):519–26.

45. Edge, R. and Navon, S. Scleral perforation during retrobulbar and peribulbar anesthesia: Risk factors and outcome in 50,000 consecutive injections. *J Cataract Refract Surg* 1999;25(9):1237–44.

46. Gadkari, S. S. Evaluation of 19 cases of inadvertent globe perforation due to periocular injections. *Indian J Ophthalmol* 2007;55(2):103–7.

47. Frieman, B. J. and Friedberg, M. A. Globe perforation associated with subtenon's anesthesia. *Am J Ophthalmol* 2001;131(4):520–1.

48. Wadood, A. C., Dhillon, B. and Singh, J. Inadvertent ocular perforation and intravitreal injection of an anesthetic agent during retrobulbar injection. *J Cataract Refract Surg* 2002;28(3):562–5.
49. Minihan, M. and Williamson, T. H. Ocular explosions from periocular anesthetic injections. *Ophthalmology* 2000;107(11):1965.
50. Puri, P., Verma, D. and McKibbin, M. Management of ocular perforations resulting from peribulbar anaesthesia. *Indian J Ophthalmol* 1999;47(3):181–3.
51. McCombe, M. and Heriot, W. Penetrating ocular injury following local anaesthesia. *Aust NZ J Ophthalmol* 1995;23(1):33–6.
52. Ling, R., Cole, M., James, C. et al. Suprachoroidal haemorrhage complicating cataract surgery in the UK: Epidemiology, clinical features, management, and outcomes. *Br J Ophthalmol* 2004;88(4):478–80.
53. Speaker, M. G., Guerriero, P. N., Met, J. A. et al. A case-control study of risk factors for intraoperative suprachoroidal expulsive hemorrhage. *Ophthalmology* 1991;98(2):202–9.
54. Mahroo, O. A., Dybowski, R., Wong, R. and Williamson, T. H. Characteristics of rhegmatogenous retinal detachment in pseudophakic and phakic eyes. *Eye (Lond)* 2012;26(8):1114–21.
55. Costen, M. T., Williams, C. P., Asteriades, S. and Luff, A. J. An unusual maculopathy after routine cataract surgery. *Eye (Lond)* 2007;21(11):1416–8.

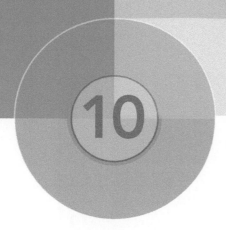

Uveitis and allied disorders

NON-INFECTIOUS UVEITIS OF THE POSTERIOR SEGMENT

There are a variety of possible presentations of uveitis of the posterior segment[1-3] which can be diagnosed on clinical features or systemic investigations. Detecting signs of inflammation in the presence of white cells in the vitreous identifies them:

- Intermediate uveitis
- Sarcoidosis
- Uveitis of juvenile chronic arthritis
- Behcet's disease
- Idiopathic vasculitis including Eales' disease
- Birdshot chorioretinopathy
- Vogt–Koyanagi–Harada syndrome
- Sympathetic uveitis
- Takayasu's arteritis (Figures 10.1 through 10.3)

In the Western population, the most common presentations are intermediate uveitis, sarcoidosis and juvenile chronic arthritis.

REFERRAL FOR VITRECTOMY

Vitrectomy is sometimes required for the following:

- Diagnostic confirmation
- Vitreous opacification
- RRD
- TRD
- Exudative RD
- CMO
- ERM
- Hypotony

Vitreous opacity occurs from white cells, cellular deposits, proteinaceous infiltration and degeneration of the gel structure. The inflammatory process can cause shrinkage of the gel, which, in the presence of vitreoretinal adhesion, will produce secondary TRD or RRD if a tear

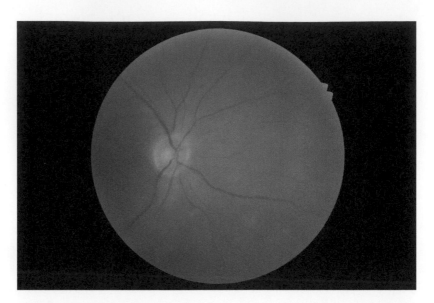

Figure 10.1 Patient with birdshot chorioretinitis.

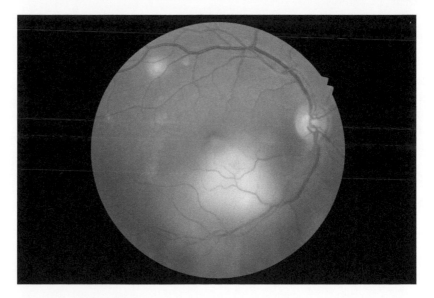

Figure 10.2 Patient with a large inflammatory lesion from sarcoidosis.

is created.[1,4,5] In patients with intermediate uveitis, CMO is a common complication seen in 40% of all eyes. Sixty per cent of eyes with poor vision have CMO.[6,7] Hypotony is a risk from the destruction of the ciliary body or traction on the ciliary body from the anterior membrane formation. Ultimately, phthisis bulbi,[8] severe shrinkage of the low-pressure eye, will be associated with complete loss of vision. The phthisical eye may be a cosmetically unacceptable eye.

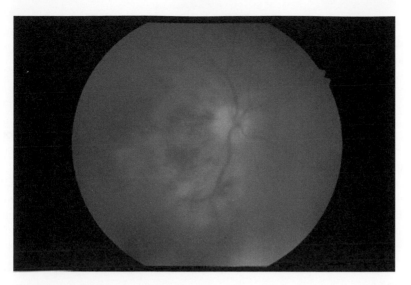

Figure 10.3 Retinal vasculitis from Behcet's disease.

VITREOUS OPACIFICATION

Vitrectomy may restore vision in patients with vitreous opacification from panuveitis.[2,9–12] Visual recovery may not be complete because of the presence of optic atrophy, retinal atrophy, retinal ischaemia or CMO.[13,14] The removal of the gel may reduce the ability of the eye to hold inflammatory mediators and, thereby, reduce the recurrence of inflammation in the long term. However, evidence for this remains uncertain.[1,4]

Retinal vasculitis produces ischaemia of the retina, which may respond by producing neo-vascularisation, which risks VH or TRD. Referral for PPV can be considered to do the following:

- Relieve traction
- Clear the visual axis[15]

RETINAL DETACHMENT

- TRD is caused by neovascularisation or fibrosis but may be accompanied by severe subretinal exudation.
- RRD may occur from PVD formation or traction and should be referred urgently.
- Exudative RD, a rare complication, may be encountered and diagnosed by shifting fluid, the absence of retinal tears, traction or epiretinal fibrosis (despite a long-standing duration of RD).[16] If immunosuppressive therapy does not reattach the retina, occasionally, vitrectomy may be considered for drainage of the exudative fluid.

CYSTOID MACULAR OEDEMA

Apart from systemic therapy, steroid can be administered locally to the eye by the following:

- Intravitreal injections
- Intravitreal implants
- Sub-Tenon's injection
- Orbital floor injection

Table 10.1 Non-infectious uveitis

Condition	Referral	Why?
Non-infectious uveitis	If undiagnosed, needs emergency referral	Needs investigation to ascertain the diagnosis

CMO often returns after a few months[17] because of the chronic nature of most cases of uveitis. The slow release dexamethasone pellets can be injected as an outpatient procedure and have an effect for 3–6 months.[18,19]

PPV has been performed to try to relieve the traction on the macula to resolve CMO[7,13,20] because the vitreous is often attached in these patients. Its effectiveness remains uncertain[21] with both improvement[5,22] and persistence of CMO described following vitrectomy.[23,24] Separating the response to vitrectomy from the natural history of the condition and from the effects of concomitant therapies is difficult.

HYPOTONY

Low IOP (hypotony) occurs because the uveitic process damages the ciliary body or because the traction from ERMs separates the ciliary processes from the choroid (Table 10.1).

The following are the causes of ciliary body failure:

- Traction
- Atrophy
- Detachment

The following are the treatments:

- Vitrectomy to try to relieve traction on the ciliary body in hypotony[11]
- Insertion of viscoelastic fluid into the anterior chamber to provide a temporary IOP rise
- Silicone oil for a more prolonged effect and to prevent severe shrinkage of the size of the eye if hypotony persists[25] and phthisis bulbi is imminent

INFECTIOUS UVEITIS

ACUTE RETINAL NECROSIS

CLINICAL FEATURES

Viral infections of the retina cause a mixed arteritic, ischaemic and infiltrative retinitis. The most common viruses involved are from the herpes simplex family[26]:

- Herpes simplex 1 is more common in the young age group.[27,28] These patients often have a history of cold sores.
- Herpes zoster is more common in the elderly[29–31] and can be associated with herpes zoster ophthalmicus[32–34] and chicken pox.[35]
- Herpes simplex 2 infections can occur especially in children.[27,36,37]
- Epstein–Barr virus (EBV) can be detected in vitreous samples but is often considered to be coincidental.[33]

Table 10.2 Acute retinal necrosis

Condition	Referral	Why?
Acute retinal necrosis	Emergency for biopsy and diagnosis	Immediate antiviral therapy is required

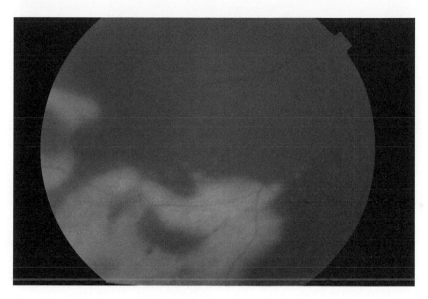

Figure 10.4 Area of retina with acute retinal necrosis.

Patients are generally not immune compromised. Progressive outer retinal necrosis is a rare and a very severe form of viral retinitis in acquired immune deficiency syndrome (AIDS) patients[38–43] and immune-compromised patients with minimal inflammatory signs.

In acute retinal necrosis (ARN), there is a high risk of bilateral disease[44,45] with fellow eye involvement even years later[46] and a long-term risk of viral encephalitis (Table 10.2).[47,48]

In ARN, the retina has the appearance of peripheral retinal haemorrhage and infiltration, which progress posteriorly eventually involving the macula and optic nerve.[48] The retina may become 'moth-eaten', and RD is common, occurring in 50%.[49] Oxidative RD is possible.[50] Patients may have GRTs,[51] retinal neovascularisation[52] and peripheral retinal pigment epithelial tears.[53] PVR in particular is very common.

Referral of a suspected case should be performed as an emergency because early intervention before the retinitis reaches the posterior retina has better outcomes (Figure 10.4).

CYTOMEGALOVIRUS RETINITIS

CLINICAL FEATURES

Cytomegalovirus (CMV) infects the retina in immune-compromised patients especially patients with AIDS. Prior to the availability of highly active antiretroviral therapy (HAART),[54] CMV retinitis developed in 40% of AIDS patients. Any patients with systemic immunesuppression such as Wegener's granulomatosis or rheumatoid arthritis are at risk.[26,55] In AIDS, the

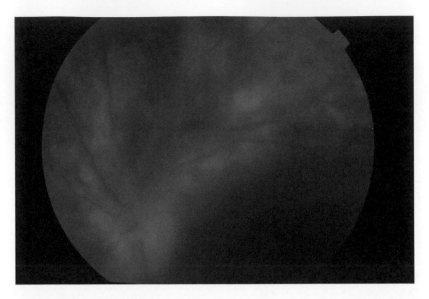

Figure 10.5 Retina with CMV infection.

patient usually has a severe reduction in CD4 white blood cells, less than 50 cells/μL. With the introduction of HAART, the control of viral load is much improved, and consequently, CD4 counts are more often preserved, leading to a large reduction in the numbers of new cases of retinitis. Failure of, or resistance to, HAART[56–59] may allow CMV retinitis.

RD is a common complication of the retinitis (50% at 1 year after development of retinitis[54,60]), usually slow in onset and progression because of the presence of a formed and attached vitreous gel in these young patients and bilateral in 70%[61] (Figure 10.5).

Without HAART, patients with CMV retinitis had poor survival of approximately 6 months.[62,63] With HAART, patients with CMV retinitis have shown an 81% reduction in mortality[64] and a 60% reduction in RD.[65]

Immune recovery uveitis and inflammatory response to the infection can reduce vision,[66–68] characterised by posterior segment inflammation and CMO,[63] vitreomacular traction,[69] VH from retinal neovascularisation[70] and activation of previously quiescent infections of the retina such as mycobacteria.[71] Immune recovery uveitis is usually self-limiting, causing only mild visual loss. Control of the viral load is used to control the retinitis, allowing the cessation of anti-CMV therapy as the CD4 count recovers.[70]

Visual Outcome

If RD complicates CMV retinitis, visual recovery is better when the retina can be fixed with one operation,[72] and good vision is possible in only approximately 50% (Table 10.3).[73]

Table 10.3 CMV retinitis

Condition	Referral	Why?
CMV retinitis	Emergency for biopsy and diagnosis	Immediate antiviral therapy is required

FUNGAL ENDOPHTHALMITIS

CLINICAL FEATURES

Fungal endophthalmitis (predominantly *Candida albicans*) is seen in patients with intravenous long lines[74,75] (e.g. patients in intensive care units) or in patients with a history of intravenous drug abuse such as heroin or crystal meth.[76] A slowly progressive endophthalmitis occurs, occasionally bilateral,[77] commencing with a white spot on the retina and then preretinal puff ball infiltration (string of pearls). It may be seen on the screening of patients in intensive care in an otherwise visually asymptomatic patient.[76,78] An intravenous line may have been used on only one occasion in order to introduce the infection[79] (Figures 10.6 and 10.7).

Infections have been reported in the following:

- Gynaecological procedures[80,81]
- Toxic megacolon[82]
- Post-partum[83,84]
- Premature infants[85–87]
- Contaminated infusion fluid in cataract extraction[88]
- Penetrating injury,[89] e.g. in a hop grower[90]

In heroin abuse, the patient presents with a reduction of vision after using acidic agents such as lemon juice (infected with Candida) to dissolve brown heroin.

Infection progresses to a more severe vitreal infiltration with typical 'string of pearl' (puff-balls) often with aggregations of white cells on the retina if the vitreous is detached. There may

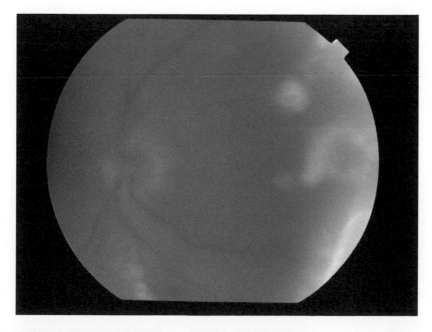

Figure 10.6 Hazy vitreous and intravitreal puff balls in Candida infection.

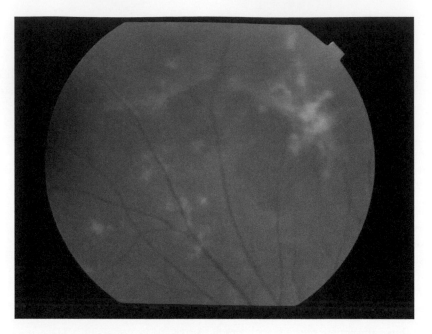

Figure 10.7 Patient with Candida infection of the eye.

be one or more foci of infiltration in the retina and choroid at the posterior pole. The following are the complications:

- ERMs are common[91]
- RD
- Phthisis bulbi[88]

The following are the infective agents:

- *Candida albicans* common
- Others, such as *Candida krusei*,[92] rarely
- 15% of cases involve aspergillus
- Fusarium rarely[93]

Visual Outcome

Visual recovery depends on the duration and severity of the infection and the location of any chorioretinal foci. Results can be good if the infection is dealt with promptly. Visual recovery with endophthalmitis caused by aspergillus is usually poor (Table 10.4).

Table 10.4 Fungal endophthalmitis

Condition	Referral	Why?
Fungal endophthalmitis	Emergency for biopsy and diagnosis	Immediate antifungal therapy and vitrectomy is required

OTHER INFECTIONS

- Toxoplasmosis is associated with RDs in approximately 6% of cases. Vitrectomy may be necessary to clear out vitreous debris or to treat secondary RD or ERM (Figures 10.8 and 10.9).
- *Toxocara canis* is very rare but can cause TRDs in childhood.
- Tuberculosis produces a vasculitis with a risk of RD despite response to systemic therapy.

Vitrectomy can be used to try to ascertain the diagnosis in infectious uveitis.

The causes of vitritis detectable by polymerase chain reaction are as follows:

- Herpes simplex viruses 1 and 2
- Varicella zoster virus
- CMV
- EBV

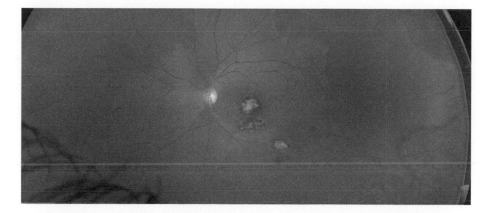

Figure 10.8 Old inactive toxoplasmosis scars.

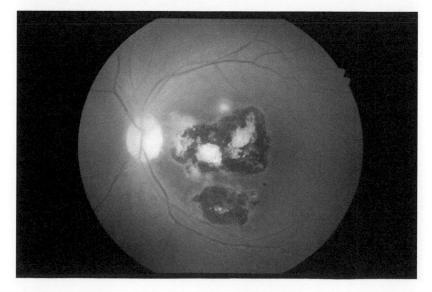

Figure 10.9 Toxoplasmosis in the macula.

- *Borrelia burgdorferi*
- *Toxoplasma gondii*
- *Mycobacterium tuberculosis*
- *Propionibacterium acnes*
- Whipple's disease

OCULAR LYMPHOMA

CLINICAL FEATURES

Lymphoma of the eye presents in the elderly, female and bilaterally.[94] Ocular lymphoma should be considered in any older patient with posterior uveitis.[95] The clinical features include intra-vitreal white cells in an otherwise quiet eye. There may be subretinal infiltration and occasionally haemorrhagic retinal necrosis.[96,97] Pseudohypopyon may be seen.[98] Fifty per cent of cases present with ocular symptoms or signs. Fifty per cent develop central nervous system (CNS) involvement first (20% of CNS lymphoma will affect the eye).[95,99] Usually, a diffused large cell B-cell lymphoma is implicated.[100]

The patient needs referral for investigation for systemic or intracerebral lymphoma. Low-dose radiotherapy to the eyes has been used.[101] Vitrectomy can be used to help provide samples for histological diagnosis and to improve vision. Systemic chemotherapy may be used (Figure 10.10).[96]

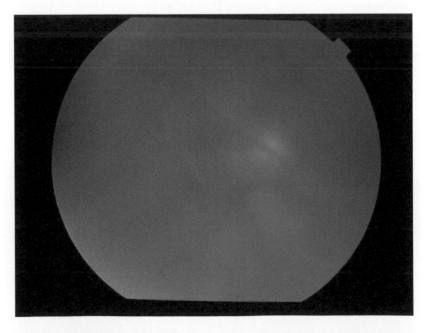

Figure 10.10 Hazy vitreous in a patient with lymphoma.

Table 10.5 Ocular lymphoma

Condition	Referral	Why?
Ocular lymphoma	Urgently for biopsy and diagnosis	Treatment may improve the vision; intracranial lymphoma needs to be investigated

VISUAL OUTCOME AND SURVIVAL

The prognosis for visual recovery is generally good. Although the lymphomas do not usually spread systemically, these patients have a shortened life expectancy due to the development of CNS lymphoma. Survival is a median of 3 years (Table 10.5).[102]

PARANEOPLASTIC RETINOPATHY

Patients with systemic carcinoma or melanoma may present with severe loss of vision with a non-specific panuveitis[103] caused by antibodies to the retina. Loss of vision occurs centrally with scotoma and photopsia. There are diffused non-specific retinal changes in the presence of severe loss of vision.

REFERENCES

1. Mieler, W. F., Will, B. R., Lewis, H. and Aaberg, T. M. Vitrectomy in the management of peripheral uveitis. *Ophthalmology* 1988;95(7):859–64.
2. Eckardt, C. and Bacskulin, A. Vitrectomy in intermediate uveitis. *Dev Ophthalmol* 1992;23:232–8.
3. Nolle, B. and Eckardt, C. Vitrectomy in multifocal chorioretinitis. *Ger J Ophthalmol* 1993;2(1):14–9.
4. Bovey, E. H. and Herbort, C. P. Vitrectomy in the management of uveitis. *Ocul Immunol Inflamm* 2000;8(4):285–91.
5. Heiligenhaus, A., Bornfeld, N., Foerster, M. H. and Wessing, A. Long-term results of pars plana vitrectomy in the management of complicated uveitis. *Br J Ophthalmol* 1994;78(7):549–54.
6. Scott, R. A., Haynes, R. J., Orr, G. M. et al. Vitreous surgery in the management of chronic endogenous posterior uveitis. *Eye* 2003;17(2):221–7.
7. Dugel, P. U., Rao, N. A., Ozler, S. et al. Pars plana vitrectomy for intraocular inflammation-related cystoid macular edema unresponsive to corticosteroids: A preliminary study. *Ophthalmology* 1992;99(10):1535–41.
8. Kokame, G. T., de Leon, M. D. and Tanji, T. Serous retinal detachment and cystoid macular edema in hypotony maculopathy. *Am J Ophthalmol* 2001;131(3):384–6.
9. Mieler, W. F. and Aaberg, T. M. Vitreous surgery in the management of peripheral uveitis. *Dev Ophthalmol* 1992;23:239–50.
10. Heimann, K., Schmanke, L., Brunner, R. and Amerian, B. Pars plana vitrectomy in the treatment of chronic uveitis. *Dev Ophthalmol* 1992;23:196–203.
11. Kaplan, H. J. Surgical treatment of intermediate uveitis. *Dev Ophthalmol* 1992;23:185–9.
12. Diamond, J. G. and Kaplan, H. J. Uveitis: Effect of vitrectomy combined with lensectomy. *Ophthalmology* 1979;86(7):1320–9.

13. Verbraeken, H. Therapeutic pars plana vitrectomy for chronic uveitis: A retrospective study of the long-term results. *Graefes Arch Clin Exp Ophthalmol* 1996;234(5):288–93.
14. Waters, F. M., Goodall, K., Jones, N. P. and McLeod, D. Vitrectomy for vitreous opacification in Fuchs' heterochromic uveitis. *Eye* 2000;14(Pt 2):216–8.
15. Potter, M. J., Myckatyn, S. O., Maberley, A. L. and Lee, A. S. Vitrectomy for pars planitis complicated by vitreous hemorrhage: Visual outcome and long-term follow-up. *Am J Ophthalmol* 2001;131(4):514–5.
16. Gaun, S., Kurimoto, Y., Komurasaki, Y. and Yoshimura, N. Vitreous surgery for bilateral bullous retinal detachment in Vogt–Koyanagi–Harada syndrome. *Ophthalmic Surg Lasers* 2002;33(6):508–10.
17. Antcliffe, R. J., Spalton, D. J., Stanford, M. R. et al. Intravitreal triamcinolone for uveitic cystoid macular oedema: An optical coherence tomography study. *Ophthalmology* 2001;108:765–2.
18. Haller, J. A., Bandello, F., Belfort, R. Jr. et al. Randomized, sham-controlled trial of dexamethasone intravitreal implant in patients with macular edema due to retinal vein occlusion. *Ophthalmology* 2010;117(6):1134–46.e3.
19. Haller, J. A., Kuppermann, B. D., Blumenkranz, M. S. et al. Randomized controlled trial of an intravitreous dexamethasone drug delivery system in patients with diabetic macular edema. *Arch Ophthalmol* 2010;128(3):289–96.
20. Aylward, G. W. The place of vitreoretinal surgery in the treatment of macular oedema. *Doc Ophthalmol* 1999;97(3–4):433–8.
21. Davis, J. L., Chan, C. C. and Nussenblatt, R. B. Diagnostic vitrectomy in intermediate uveitis. *Dev Ophthalmol* 1992;23:120–32.
22. Tranos, P., Scott, R., Zambarakji, H. et al. The effect of pars plana vitrectomy on cystoid macular oedema associated with chronic uveitis: A randomised, controlled pilot study. *Br J Ophthalmol* 2006;90(9):1107–10.
23. Diamond, J. G. and Kaplan, H. J. Lensectomy and vitrectomy for complicated cataract secondary to uveitis. *Arch Ophthalmol* 1978;96(10):1798–804.
24. Priem, H., Verbraeken, H. and De Laey, J. J. Diagnostic problems in chronic vitreous inflammation. *Graefes Arch Clin Exp Ophthalmol* 1993;231(8):453–6.
25. Morse, L. S. and McCuen, B. W. The use of silicone oil in uveitis and hypotony. *Retina* 1991;11(4):399–404.
26. Akpek, E. K., Kent, C., Jakobiec, F. et al. Bilateral acute retinal necrosis caused by cytomegalovirus in an immunocompromised patient. *Am J Ophthalmol* 1999;127(1):93–5.
27. Rahhal, F. M., Siegel, L. M., Russak, V. et al. Clinicopathologic correlations in acute retinal necrosis caused by herpes simplex virus type 2. *Arch Ophthalmol* 1996;114(11):1416–9.
28. Lewis, M. L., Culbertson, W. W., Post, J. D. et al. Herpes simplex virus type 1: A cause of the acute retinal necrosis syndrome. *Ophthalmology* 1989;96(6):875–8.
29. Freeman, W. R., Thomas, E. L., Rao, N. A. et al. Demonstration of herpes group virus in acute retinal necrosis syndrome. *Am J Ophthalmol* 1986;102(6):701–9.
30. Bali, E., Huyghe, P., Caspers, L. and Libert, J. Vitrectomy and silicone oil in the treatment of acute endophthalmitis: Preliminary results. *Bull Soc Belge Ophtalmol* 2003(288):9–14.
31. Zambarakji, H. J., Obi, A. A. and Mitchell, S. M. Successful treatment of varicella zoster virus retinitis with aggressive intravitreal and systemic antiviral therapy. *Ocul Immunol Inflamm* 2002;10(1):41–6.
32. Nakanishi, F., Takahashi, H. and Ohara, K. Acute retinal necrosis following contralateral herpes zoster ophthalmicus. *Jpn J Ophthalmol* 2000;44(5):561–4.

33. Hershberger, V. S., Hutchins, R. K., Witte, D. P. et al. Epstein–Barr virus-related bilateral acute retinal necrosis in a patient with X-linked lymphoproliferative disorder. *Arch Ophthalmol* 2003;121(7):1047–9.

34. Weinberg, D. V. and Lyon, A. T. Repair of retinal detachments due to herpes varicella-zoster virus retinitis in patients with acquired immune deficiency syndrome. *Ophthalmology* 1997;104(2):279–82.

35. Culbertson, W. W., Brod, R. D., Flynn, H. W. Jr. et al. Chickenpox-associated acute retinal necrosis syndrome. *Ophthalmology* 1991;98(11):1641–5.

36. Markomichelakis, N. N., Zafirakis, P., Karambogia-Karefillidi, P. et al. Herpes simplex virus type 2: A cause of acute retinal necrosis syndrome. *Ocul Immunol Inflamm* 2001;9(2):103–9.

37. Rappaport, K. D. and Tang, W. M. Herpes simplex virus type 2 acute retinal necrosis in a patient with systemic lupus erythematosus. *Retina* 2000;20(5):545–6.

38. Purdy, K. W., Heckenlively, J. R., Church, J. A. and Keller, M. A. Progressive outer retinal necrosis caused by varicella-zoster virus in children with acquired immunodeficiency syndrome. *Pediatr Infect Dis J* 2003;22(4):384–6.

39. Austin, R. B. Progressive outer retinal necrosis syndrome: A comprehensive review of its clinical presentation, relationship to immune system status, and management. *Clin Eye Vis Care* 2000;12(3–4):119–29.

40. Moorthy, R. S., Weinberg, D. V., Teich, S. A. et al. Management of varicella zoster virus retinitis in AIDS. *Br J Ophthalmol* 1997;81(3):189–94.

41. Perez-Blazquez, E., Traspas, R., Mendez, M. I. and Montero, M. Intravitreal ganciclovir treatment in progressive outer retinal necrosis. *Am J Ophthalmol* 1997;124(3):418–21.

42. Pavesio, C. E., Mitchell, S. M., Barton, K. et al. Progressive outer retinal necrosis (PORN) in AIDS patients: A different appearance of varicella-zoster retinitis. *Eye* 1995;9 (Pt 3):271–6.

43. Margolis, T. P., Lowder, C. Y., Holland, G. N. et al. Varicella-zoster virus retinitis in patients with the acquired immunodeficiency syndrome. *Am J Ophthalmol* 1991;112(2):119–31.

44. Ezra, E., Pearson, R. V., Etchells, D. E. and Gregor, Z. J. Delayed fellow eye involvement in acute retinal necrosis syndrome. *Am J Ophthalmol* 1995;120(1):115–7.

45. Martinez, J., Lambert, H. M., Capone, A. et al. Delayed bilateral involvement in the acute retinal necrosis syndrome. *Am J Ophthalmol* 1992;113(1):103–4.

46. Matsuo, T., Nakayama, T., Koyama, T. and Matsuo, N. Mild type acute retinal necrosis syndrome involving both eyes at three-year interval. *Jpn J Ophthalmol* 1987;31(3):455–60.

47. Ahmadieh, H., Sajjadi, S. H., Azarmina, M. and Kalani, H. Association of herpetic encephalitis with acute retinal necrosis syndrome. *Ann Ophthalmol* 1991;23(6):215–9.

48. Bloom, J. N., Katz, J. I. and Kaufman, H. E. Herpes simplex retinitis and encephalitis in an adult. *Arch Ophthalmol* 1977;95(10):1798–9.

49. Carney, M. D., Peyman, G. A., Goldberg, M. F. et al. Acute retinal necrosis. *Retina* 1986;6(2):85–94.

50. Duker, J. S., Nielsen, J. C., Eagle, R. C. Jr. et al. Rapidly progressive acute retinal necrosis secondary to herpes simplex virus, type 1. *Ophthalmology* 1990;97(12):1638–43.

51. Topilow, H. W., Nussbaum, J. J., Freeman, H. M. et al. Bilateral acute retinal necrosis: Clinical and ultrastructural study. *Arch Ophthalmol* 1982;100(12):1901–8.

52. Wang, C. L., Kaplan, H. J., Waldrep, J. C. and Pulliam, M. Retinal neovascularization associated with acute retinal necrosis. *Retina* 1983;3(4):249–52.

53. Fox, G. M. and Blumenkranz, M. Giant retinal pigment epithelial tears in acute retinal necrosis. *Am J Ophthalmol* 1993;116(3):302–6.

54. Jabs, D. A. Ocular manifestations of HIV infection. *Trans Am Ophthalmol Soc* 1995;93:623–83.

55. Fraenkel, G., Ross, B. and Wong, H. C. Cytomegalovirus retinitis in a patient with rheumatoid arthritis being treated with combination immunosuppressive therapy. *Retina* 1995;15(2):169–70.

56. Uphold, C. R., Smith, M. F. and Bender, B. S. Failure of a prospective trial to detect cytomegalovirus retinitis after initiation of highly active antiretroviral therapy. *AIDS Patient Care STDS* 1998;12(12):907–12.

57. Mitchell, S. M., Membrey, W. L., Youle, M. S. et al. Cytomegalovirus retinitis after the initiation of highly active antiretroviral therapy: A 2 year prospective study. *Br J Ophthalmol* 1999;83(6):652–5.

58. Mocroft, A., Katlama, C., Johnson, A. M. et al. AIDS across Europe, 1994–98: The EuroSIDA study. *Lancet* 2000;356(9226):291–6.

59. Jalali, S., Reed, J. B., Mizoguchi, M. et al. Effect of highly active antiretroviral therapy on the incidence of HIV-related cytomegalovirus retinitis and retinal detachment. *AIDS Patient Care STDS* 2000;14(7):343–6.

60. Jabs, D. A., Enger, C., Haller, J. and de Bustros, S. Retinal detachments in patients with cytomegalovirus retinitis. *Arch Ophthalmol* 1991;109(6):794–9.

61. Sidikaro, Y., Silver, L., Holland, G. N. and Kreiger, A. E. Rhegmatogenous retinal detachments in patients with AIDS and necrotizing retinal infections. *Ophthalmology* 1991;98(2):129–35.

62. Dugel, P. U., Liggett, P. E., Lee, M. B. et al. Repair of retinal detachment caused by cytomegalovirus retinitis in patients with the acquired immunodeficiency syndrome. *Am J Ophthalmol* 1991;112(3):235–42.

63. Irvine, A. R., Lonn, L., Schwartz, D. et al. Retinal detachment in AIDS: Long-term results after repair with silicone oil. *Br J Ophthalmol* 1997;81(3):180–3.

64. Kempen, J. H., Jabs, D. A., Wilson, L. A. et al. Mortality risk for patients with cytomegalovirus retinitis and acquired immune deficiency syndrome. *Clin Infect Dis* 2003;37(10):1365–73.

65. Kempen, J. H., Jabs, D. A., Dunn, J. P. et al. Retinal detachment risk in cytomegalovirus retinitis related to the acquired immunodeficiency syndrome. *Arch Ophthalmol* 2001;119(1):33–40.

66. Holbrook, J. T., Jabs, D. A., Weinberg, D. V. et al. Visual loss in patients with cytomegalovirus retinitis and acquired immunodeficiency syndrome before widespread availability of highly active antiretroviral therapy. *Arch Ophthalmol* 2003;121(1):99–107.

67. Arevalo, J. F., Mendoza, A. J. and Ferretti, Y. Immune recovery uveitis in AIDS patients with cytomegalovirus retinitis treated with highly active antiretroviral therapy in Venezuela. *Retina* 2003;23(4):495–502.

68. Song, M. K., Azen, S. P., Buley, A. et al. Effect of anti-cytomegalovirus therapy on the incidence of immune recovery uveitis in AIDS patients with healed cytomegalovirus retinitis. *Am J Ophthalmol* 2003;136(4):696–702.

69. Canzano, J. C., Reed, J. B. and Morse, L. S. Vitreomacular traction syndrome following highly active antiretroviral therapy in AIDS patients with cytomegalovirus retinitis. *Retina* 1998;18(5):443–7.

70. Wright, M. E., Suzman, D. L., Csaky, K. G. et al. Extensive retinal neovascularization as a late finding in human immunodeficiency virus-infected patients with immune recovery uveitis. *Clin Infect Dis* 2003;36(8):1063–6.

71. Zamir, E., Hudson, H., Ober, R. R. et al. Massive mycobacterial choroiditis during highly active antiretroviral therapy: Another immune-recovery uveitis? *Ophthalmology* 2002;109(11):2144–8.

72. Scott, I. U., Flynn, H. W., Lai, M. et al. First operation anatomic success and other predictors of postoperative vision after complex retinal detachment repair with vitrectomy and silicone oil tamponade. *Am J Ophthalmol* 2000;130(6):745–50.

73. Azen, S. P., Scott, I. U., Flynn, H. W. Jr. et al. Silicone oil in the repair of complex retinal detachments. A prospective observational multicenter study. *Ophthalmology* 1998;105(9):1587–97.

74. Graham, E., Chignell, A. H. and Eykyn, S. Candida endophthalmitis: A complication of prolonged intravenous therapy and antibiotic treatment. *J Infect* 1986;13(2):167–73.

75. Jackson, T. L., Eykyn, S. J., Graham, E. M. and Stanford, M. R. Endogenous bacterial endophthalmitis: A 17-year prospective series and review of 267 reported cases. *Surv Ophthalmol* 2003;48(4):403–23.

76. Aguilar, G. L., Blumenkrantz, M. S., Egbert, P. R. and McCulley, J. P. Candida endophthalmitis after intravenous drug abuse. *Arch Ophthalmol* 1979;97(1):96–100.

77. Wong, V. K., Tasman, W., Eagle, R. C. Jr. and Rodriguez, A. Bilateral *Candida parapsilosis* endophthalmitis. *Arch Ophthalmol* 1997;115(5):670–2.

78. Chignell, A. H. Endogenous Candida endophthalmitis. *J R Soc Med* 1992;85(12):721–4.

79. Gupta, A., Gupta, V., Dogra, M. R. et al. Fungal endophthalmitis after a single intravenous administration of presumably contaminated dextrose infusion fluid. *Retina* 2000;20(3):262–8.

80. Chang, T. S., Chen, W. C., Chen, H. S. and Lee, H. W. Endogenous *Candida* endophthalmitis after two consecutive procedures of suction dilatation and curettage. *Chang Gung Med J* 2002;25(11):778–82.

81. Chen, S. J., Chung, Y. M. and Liu, J. H. Endogenous *Candida* endophthalmitis after induced abortion. *Am J Ophthalmol* 1998;125(6):873–5.

82. Henderson, T. and Irfan, S. Bilateral endogenous *Candida* endophthalmitis and chorioretinitis following toxic megacolon. *Eye* 1996;10 (Pt 6):755–7.

83. Tsai, C. C., Chen, S. J., Chung, Y. M. et al. Postpartum endogenous *Candida* endophthalmitis. *J Formos Med Assoc* 2002;101(6):432–6.

84. Cantrill, H. L., Rodman, W. P., Ramsay, R. C. and Knobloch, W. H. Postpartum *Candida* endophthalmitis. *JAMA* 1980;243(11):1163–5.

85. Gago, L. C., Capone, A. Jr. and Trese, M. T. Bilateral presumed endogenous Candida endophthalmitis and stage 3 retinopathy of prematurity. *Am J Ophthalmol* 2002; 134(4):611–3.

86. Stern, J. H., Calvano, C. and Simon, J. W. Recurrent endogenous candidal endophthalmitis in a premature infant. *JAAPOS* 2001;5(1):50–1.

87. Annable, W. L., Kachmer, M. L., DiMarco, M. and DeSantis, D. Long-term follow-up of Candida endophthalmitis in the premature infant. *J Pediatr Ophthalmol Strabismus* 1990;27(2):103–6.

88. Sasoh, M., Uji, Y., Arima, M. et al. Retinal detachment due to breaks in pars plicata of ciliary body after endogenous fungal endophthalmitis. *Jpn J Ophthalmol* 1993;37(1):93–9.

89. Peyman, G. A., Vastine, D. W. and Diamond, J. G. Vitrectomy in exogenous Candida endophthalmitis. *Albrecht Von Graefes Arch Klin Exp Ophthalmol* 1975;197(1):55–9.

90. Mackiewicz, J., Haszcz, D. and Zagorski, Z. Exogenous *Candida* endophthalmitis in a hop grower – A case report. *Ann Agric Environ Med* 2000;7(2):131–2.

91. McDonald, H. R., de Bustros, S. and Sipperley, J. O. Vitrectomy for epiretinal membrane with *Candida* chorioretinitis. *Ophthalmology* 1990;97(4):466–9.

92. McQuillen, D. P., Zingman, B. S., Meunier, F. and Levitz, S. M. Invasive infections due to *Candida krusei*: Report of ten cases of fungemia that include three cases of endophthalmitis. *Clin Infect Dis* 1992;14(2):472–8.

93. Essman, T. F., Flynn, H. W. Jr., Smiddy, W. E. et al. Treatment outcomes in a 10-year study of endogenous fungal endophthalmitis. *Ophthalmic Surg Lasers* 1997;28(3):185–94.

94. Palexas, G. N., Green, W. R., Goldberg, M. F. and Ding, Y. Diagnostic pars plana vitrectomy report of a 21-year retrospective study. *Trans Am Ophthalmol Soc* 1995;93:281–308.

95. Peterson, K., Gordon, K. B., Heinemann, M. H. and Deangelis, L. M. The clinical spectrum of ocular lymphoma. *Cancer* 1993;72(3):843–9.

96. Akpek, E. K., Ahmed, I., Hochberg, F. H. et al. Intraocular-central nervous system lymphoma: Clinical features, diagnosis, and outcomes. *Ophthalmology* 1999;106(9):1805–10.

97. Ridley, M. E., McDonald, H. R., Sternberg, P. Jr. et al. Retinal manifestations of ocular lymphoma (reticulum cell sarcoma). *Ophthalmology* 1992;99(7):1153–60.

98. Lobo, A., Larkin, G., Clark, B. J. et al. Pseudo-hypopyon as the presenting feature in B-cell and T-cell intraocular lymphoma. *Clin Experiment Ophthalmol* 2003;31(2):155–8.

99. Herrlinger, U. Primary CNS lymphoma: Findings outside the brain. *JNeurooncol* 1999;43(3):227–30.

100. Coupland, S. E., Bechrakis, N. E., Anastassiou, G. et al. Evaluation of vitrectomy specimens and chorioretinal biopsies in the diagnosis of primary intraocular lymphoma in patients with Masquerade syndrome. *Graefes Arch Clin Exp Ophthalmol* 2003;241(10):860–70.

101. Margolis, L., Fraser, R., Lichter, A. and Char, D. H. The role of radiation therapy in the management of ocular reticulum cell sarcoma. *Cancer* 1980;45(4):688–92.

102. Batara, J. F. and Grossman, S. A. Primary central nervous system lymphomas. *Curr Opin Neurol* 2003;16(6):671–5.

103. Lu, Y., Jia, L., He, S. et al. Melanoma-associated retinopathy: A paraneoplastic autoimmune complication. *Arch Ophthalmol* 2009;127(12):1572–80.

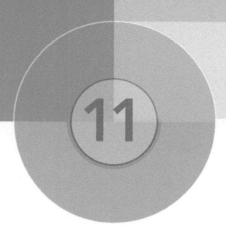

Miscellaneous conditions

VITRECTOMY FOR VITREOUS OPACITIES

Symptomatic vitreous floaters are common over the age of 30 years but are mostly ignored by the individual. Some have considerable debris in the vitreous either from pathology or from general degeneration. Some individuals do not tolerate even small floaters often related to their personality types or to activities that they perform. Patients with multifocal lens implants may find vitreous opacities more problematic.

The following are the common causes of floaters:

- PVD
- Vitreous syneresis, e.g. high myopia
- Resolved VH
- Uveitis
- Asteroid hyalosis
- Silicone oil emulsion

It is important to discriminate floaters from scotoma, the former changing position in the visual field during eye movements, while the latter is always in the same position relative to fixation. It is reassuring to detect vitreous opacities on ophthalmoscopy before offering surgery but sometimes this cannot be achieved. Watch out for previously undiagnosed conditions such as intermediate uveitis. The vitreous does not need to be detached, but a detached vitreous will be easier to remove surgically. Use OCT to look for partial detachment or to confirm the attachment of the vitreous to the optic disc. An attached vitreous means an increase in the chance of complications such as retinal tear formation, macular ERM or hole formation and VH or more likelihood for gas insertion. Overall complications have been described in 2%.[1-3] Patients are however very pleased to have no floaters after successful surgery. The removal of the vitreous opacities has been shown to improve contrast sensitivity and visual acuity. YAG vitreolysis may be able to reduce some floaters but often needs repeated treatments and has a high rate of conversion to vitrectomy but does avoid the risk of post-operative cataract formation if successful.[4]

VITREOUS ANOMALIES

PERSISTENT HYPERPLASTIC PRIMARY VITREOUS

The most frequent severe developmental anomaly in the vitreous is persistent hyperplastic primary vitreous. This is caused by a vascular structure which should regress during early development of the eye but which remains. In infancy, this may cause microphthalmic strabismic eye with leukocoria. The fibrovascular tissue invades the lens posteriorly and ultimately causes a complete cataract and secondary angle closure glaucoma. In less severe cases, vitrectomy can be used but often with little visual recovery.[5]

ASTEROID HYALOSIS

Asteroid hyalosis is a specific form of gel degeneration in which globules of calcium soaps (possibly hydroxylapatite, calcium and phosphate) aggregate on vitreous fibrils.[6] It has been found in 2% of autopsy specimens,[7] with increased prevalence with increasing age. The process of formation may be similar to lithiasis, stone formation in the body, e.g. the kidneys. Usually, they are surprisingly asymptomatic. Asteroid is not associated with any systemic condition, and the aetiology is unknown (Table 11.1). A few patients will be symptomatic, in which case, vitrectomy is required to improve vision (Figure 11.1).[8–10]

Table 11.1 Asteroid hyalosis

Condition	Referral	Why?
Asteroid hyalosis	Routine	For symptomatic floaters

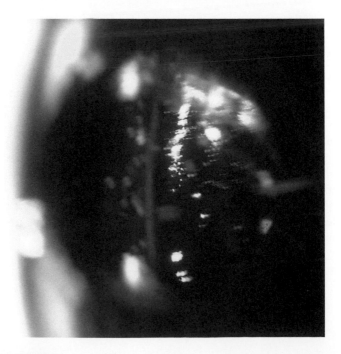

Figure 11.1 Asteroid hyalosis.

AMYLOIDOSIS

Amyloidosis of the vitreous is a very rare condition usually associated with primary or familial (dominantly inherited) forms of amyloidosis. Proteinaceous material, probably derived from the retinal circulation, becomes coated on the collagenous framework of the gel bilaterally to produce a 'glass-wool' opacification; associated cellular invasion is conspicuous by its absence.

RETINAL HAEMANGIOMA AND TELANGIECTASIA

Retinal angioma (retinal capillary haemangioma) can occur as a solitary lesion not associated with systemic disease or as multiple lesions in von Hipple–Lindau disease (VHL). Idiopathic cases present later, with mean age at presentation of 36 years, than in VHL (17 years).[11,12] Most tumours are located in the superotemporal quadrant in the retinal mid-periphery,[13] and 17% of angiomas in VHL occur on the optic nerve.[14] New tumours are rare in idiopathic cases. Isolated retinal angiomas have been described after RRD surgery[15] (Figure 11.2).

In VHL, a mean of four tumours are seen per eye, and new lesions tend to occur before the age of 47 years. In VHL, extraocular lesions occur as follows:

1. CNS haemangioma
2. Renal cyst, renal carcinoma
3. Pancreatic cysts and adenoma, pancreatic islet cell tumours
4. Phaeochromocytoma
5. Endolymphatic sac tumour of the inner ear
6. Cystadenoma of the epididymis and broad ligament

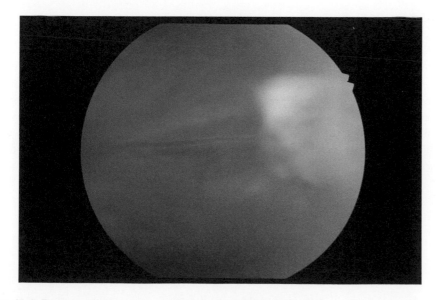

Figure 11.2 Retinal angioma in VHL showing a large feeder blood vessel.

Retinal angiomas may cause VH, tractional, exudative RD or RRD and macular pucker or hole.[16–21] Treatment may involve the following:

1. Observation
2. Laser photocoagulation of angiomas smaller than 1.5 mm
3. Cryotherapy to larger lesions
4. Vitrectomy surgery for the complications such as VH, RD and macular pucker[14,22]

Unfortunately, in RD, PVR formation is common making surgery hazardous.

External beam radiotherapy has been tried where other treatments have failed to regress the lesions.[23] An effective therapeutic option is not available for optic nerve lesions.[24]

OPTIC DISC ANOMALIES

Various optic disc anomalies are associated with retinal elevation.

OPTIC DISC PITS AND OPTIC DISC COLOBOMA

Optic disc anomalies are associated with the formation of a maculopathy consisting of intra-retinal and SRF. Theories have been postulated that the fluid arises from the disc perhaps leak-ing from the subarachnoid space or from a defect in the surface of the disc, allowing vitreous fluid to enter. The retinal elevation appears to consist of a multilayered schisis of the retina.[25] Vitrectomy and gas can be used to oppose the peripapillary retina to the RPE and allow the application of laser to seal the retina around the optic disc (Table 11.2).[26,27]

The resolution of the retinal elevation may take 9 months post-operatively.

Some patients may be suffering from renal coloboma syndrome with renal hypoplasia and a mutation of the PAX2 gene, and therefore, renal investigations may be adviseable[28] (Figures 11.3 through 11.5).

MORNING GLORY SYNDROME

This severe optic disc anomaly can be associated with posterior polar RD or schisis in as many as 35% of patients.[29] Often vision is poor because of the disc abnormality, and there is nystag-mus. A communication has been described between the subarachnoid space[30] and the subreti-nal space (metrizamide cisterography has shown dye migration into the SRF). More commonly, a hole on the optic nerve head has been blamed for the passage of fluid from the vitreous cavity to the subretinal space in a similar fashion to optic pit. For this reason, vitrectomy has been used with peripapillary laser applied to block the flow of fluid and with internal tamponade (Figure 11.6).

Table 11.2 Optic disc maculopathy

Condition	Referral	Why?
Optic disc maculopathy	Routine 1–2 months	For vitrectomy laser and gas

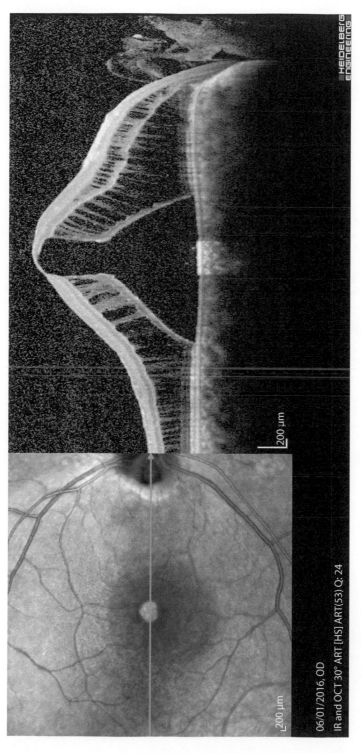

06/01/2016, OD

IR and OCT 30° ART [HS] ART(53) Q: 24

Figure 11.3 Elevation and schisis of the retina are shown in this patient with optic pit–related maculopathy.

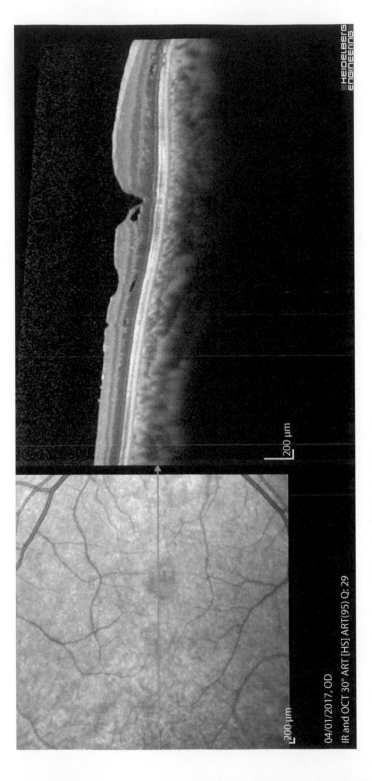

04/01/2017, OD

IR and OCT 30° ART [HS] ART(95) Q: 29

Figure 11.4 After surgery, there is resolution of the SRF and schisis cavities.

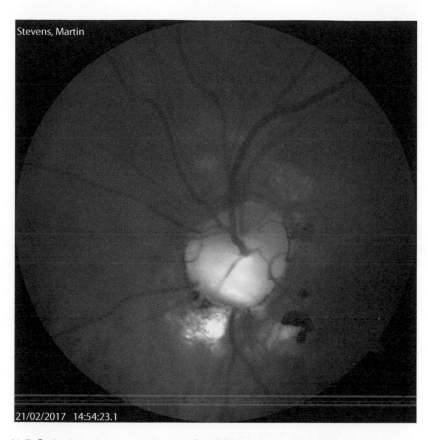

Stevens, Martin

21/02/2017   14:54:23.1

Figure 11.5 Optic disc coloboma in disorder: CHARGE syndrome. CHARGE syndrome consists of coloboma of the eye, heart defects, atresia of the choanae, retardation of growth and development and ear abnormalities and deafness.

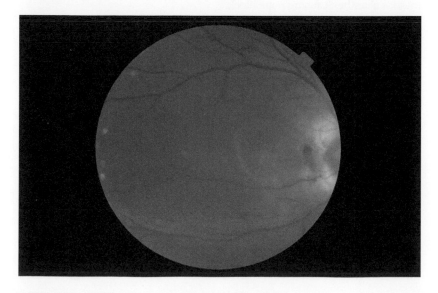

Figure 11.6 Macular elevation from a morning glory optic nerve.

RETINOCHOROIDAL COLOBOMA

Congenital coloboma of the retina and choroid can result in RRD from breaks:

- On the edge of the defect[31]
- In the coloboma[32]
- In the peripheral retina[33,34]

Vitrectomy and gas and sealing of breaks with laser can be used (Figure 11.7).

MARFAN'S SYNDROME

Marfan's syndrome is a connective tissue disorder which affects the skeleton, lungs, eyes, heart and blood vessels. The disease is characterised by unusually long limbs (arm span longer than the patient's height) and long fingers, especially the middle phalanx. Marfan's syndrome is an autosomal dominant disorder and has been linked to the FBN1 gene on chromosome 15; this encodes a protein called fibrillin, essential for the formation of elastic fibres (Figure 11.8).

These patients present in two ways with ocular problems:

- With dislocated or subluxated crystaline lenses
- With RRD associated with high myopia

The bilaterality of RRD is high at 70%[35] with tears varying from small breaks to GRTs.[36] Dislocated lenses should be removed when the edge of the lens is interfering with the visual axis. The lenses usually require removal by vitreolensectomy.[37] Lens implantation is problematic in that sutured sulcus lenses are prone to problems such as suture erosion, VH, lens tilt and dislocation in the long term.[38,39] Therefore, leaving the eye aphakic may be appropriate especially when there is high myopia, with contact lens usage thereafter. Fully dislocated lenses should be removed, as there is a risk of lens-induced uveitis or glaucoma[40] or lens dislocation into the anterior chamber, causing pupil block.

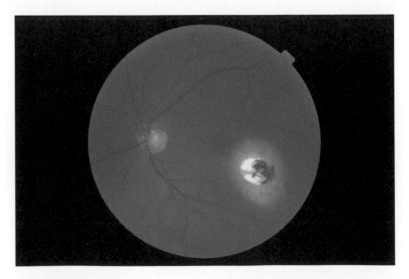

Figure 11.7 Chorioretinal coloboma.

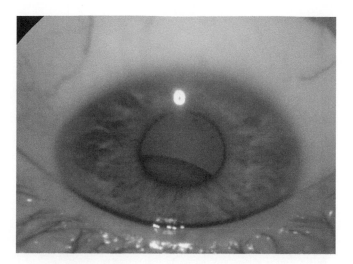

Figure 11.8 Dislocated lens in a patient with Marfan's syndrome.

RETINOPATHY OF PREMATURITY

Prematurity of birth has been defined as birth at less than 32 weeks of gestation or birth weight of less than 1500 g, but especially less than 1250 g. The retina in prematurity has not fully developed its vascularisation. This leads to ischaemia of the peripheral retina. This then leads to the development of neovascularisation of the retina secondary to the peripheral ischaemia. The eyes may progress to severe TRD and VH from neovascularisation between the vascularised and non-vascularised retina. The lowest zone and the highest stage observed in each eye categorise retinopathy of prematurity (ROP) as follows:

- Zones:
    - Zone 1: The centre of zone 1 is the optic nerve. The zone extends twice the distance from the optic nerve to the macula in a circle.
    - Zone 2: Zone 2 is a circle surrounding the zone 1 circle with the nasal ora serrata as its nasal border.
    - Zone 3: Zone 3 is the crescent that the circle of zone 2 did not encompass temporally.
- Stages:
    - Stage 0: Stage 0 is characterised by immature retinal vasculature. No clear demarcation of vascularised and non-vascularised retina is present.
    - Stage 1: A fine, thin demarcation line can be seen between the vascular and avascular regions.
    - Stage 2: A broad, thick ridge exists between the vascular and the avascular retina.
    - Stage 3: Neovascularisation is present on the ridge, on the posterior surface of the ridge or anteriorly towards the vitreous cavity.
    - Stage 4: A subtotal RD is present, beginning at the ridge.
    - Stage 4A: Stage 4A does not involve the fovea.
    - Stage 4B: Stage 4B involves the fovea.
    - Stage 5: This stage is a total RD in the shape of a funnel.
    - Stage 5A: Stage 5A is an open funnel.
    - Stage 5B: Stage 5B is a closed funnel.

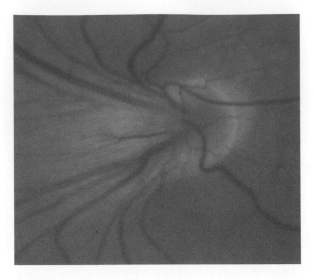

Figure 11.9 Dragged disc in a patient with previous ROP.

Plus disease is defined as the dilation and tortuosity of the peripheral retinal vessels, iris vascular engorgement, pupillary rigidity and vitreous haze.

Vitrectomy methods have been used for the more severe grades of retinopathy, stages 4A–5B. Although there are reports of patients with better vision, up to 20/25,[41] most successful anatomical outcomes result in 'fixing and following' acuities.[42–45] Functional blindness is highly likely even with surgical intervention. It has been questioned whether patients who receive vitrectomy do any better than those who have not been operated upon.[46] PPV for stage 5 ROP achieves a flat macula in only 28–45%.[47,48]

Adults who suffered ROP in infancy may present in adulthood with RRD related to myopia or early PVD. RRD occurs in early adulthood (mean: 23 years), and bilaterality is common.[49] Lattice degeneration is commonly seen,[50] and TRDs may appear. The retinas can be successfully repaired, although with a higher chance of multiple procedures of 23–50%[51–53] with final success rates of approximately 83% (Figure 11.9).

UVEAL EFFUSION SYNDROME

CLINICAL FEATURES

The uveal effusion syndrome is an unusual condition often mistaken for either a rhegmatogenous detachment complicated by choroidal detachment or a 'ring melanoma' of the anterior choroid. It is characterised by deep ciliochoroidal detachments and mottling of pigment epithelium (called *leopard spots*). Exudative RD occurs with marked 'shifting fluid' (movement of SRF with gravity) (Table 11.3). The eyes may be nanophthalmic or hypermetropic. Spontaneous resolution may occur over a period of months, but usually, they need surgery by deep excision of large patches of sclera to increase uveal–scleral outflow (Table 11.4) (Figures 11.10 and 11.11).

Table 11.3 Causes of exudative RD

Uveal effusion syndrome	
Coat's disease	
Central serous retinopathy	
Dominant exudative vitreoretinopathy	
Idiopathic telangiectasia	
Scleritis	Wegener's granulomatosis
	Rheumatoid arthritis
Endophthalmitis/cellulitis	
Uveitis	Vogt–Koyanagi–Harada syndrome
	Acute multifocal posterior pigment epitheliopathy
Vasculitis	
Tumours	Malignant melanoma
	Metastases
	Haemangioma
	VHL
Vasculopathic	Toxaemia of pregnancy
	Hypertensive retinopathy
	Ocular ischaemia
Surgery/laser	

Table 11.4 Uveal effusion syndrome

Condition	Referral	Why?
Uveal effusion syndrome	Soon	For investigation and exclusion of other pathology and then consider surgery

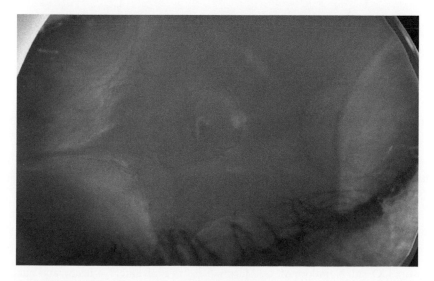

Figure 11.10 Choroidal effusions in uveal effusion syndrome.

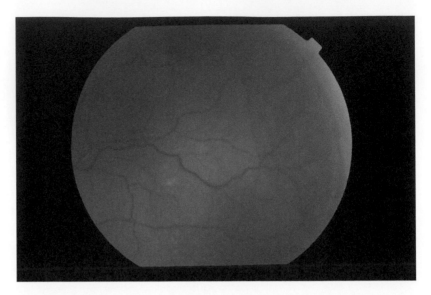

Figure 11.11 Subtle elevation of the choroid in uveal effusion syndrome.

TERSON'S SYNDROME

Patients with subarachnoid haemorrhage from intracranial aneurysms may develop vitreous bleeds.[54-60] Histopathology has shown haemorrhage in the vitreous, subhyloid, sub-ILM, intra-retinal and in the optic nerve and the optic nerve sheath. Secondary complications such as macular hole have been seen.[61] The vision can be improved by PPV surgery.[59]

DISSEMINATED INTRAVASCULAR COAGULATION

This severe presentation after septicaemia, involving widespread intravascular coagulation, resulting in loss of clotting factors, is associated with multiorgan vascular occlusion and haemorrhage. In the eye, it has been associated with choroidal infarction and VH with retinal damage and PVR.[62]

RETINAL PROSTHESIS

Retinal electrodes are being designed and trailed in patients with retinitis pigmentosa. As yet, a definitive design has not been established, but early systems have shown encouraging results for levels of vision, e.g. 16 pixels.[63,64]

REFERENCES

1. Mason, J. O. 3rd, Neimkin, M. G., Mason, J. O. 4th et al. Safety, efficacy, and quality of life following sutureless vitrectomy for symptomatic vitreous floaters. *Retina* 2014;34(6):1055–61.

2. Sebag, J., Yee, K. M., Wa, C. A. et al. Vitrectomy for floaters: Prospective efficacy analyses and retrospective safety profile. *Retina* 2014;34(6):1062–8.

3. Tan, H. S., Mura, M., Lesnik Oberstein, S. Y. and Bijl, H. M. Safety of vitrectomy for floaters. *Am J Ophthalmol* 2011;151(6):995–8.

4. Delaney, Y. M., Oyinloye, A. and Benjamin, L. Nd:YAG vitreolysis and pars plana vitrectomy: Surgical treatment for vitreous floaters. *Eye (Lond)* 2002;16(1):21–6.

5. Laatikainen, L. and Tarkkanen, A. Microsurgery of persistent hyperplastic primary vitreous. *Ophthalmologica* 1982;185(4):193–8.

6. Winkler, J. and Lunsdorf, H. Ultrastructure and composition of asteroid bodies. *Invest Ophthalmol Vis Sci* 2001;42(5):902–7.

7. Fawzi, A. A., Vo, B., Kriwanek, R. et al. Asteroid hyalosis in an autopsy population: The University of California at Los Angeles (UCLA) experience. *Arch Ophthalmol* 2005;123(4):486–90.

8. Parnes, R. E., Zakov, Z. N., Novak, M. A. and Rice, T. A. Vitrectomy in patients with decreased visual acuity secondary to asteroid hyalosis. *Am J Ophthalmol* 1998;125(5):703–4.

9. Feist, R. M., Morris, R. E., Witherspoon, C. D. et al. Vitrectomy in asteroid hyalosis. *Retina* 1990;10(3):173–7.

10. Renaldo, D. P. Pars plana vitrectomy for asteroid hyalosis. *Retina* 1981;1(3):252–4.

11. Singh, A. D., Nouri, M., Shields, C. L. et al. Retinal capillary hemangioma: A comparison of sporadic cases and cases associated with von Hippel–Lindau disease. *Ophthalmology* 2001;108(10):1907–11.

12. Singh, A., Shields, J. and Shields, C. Solitary retinal capillary hemangioma: Hereditary (von Hippel–Lindau disease) or nonhereditary? *Arch Ophthalmol* 2001;119(2):232–4.

13. Singh, A. D., Shields, C. L. and Shields, J. A. von Hippel–Lindau disease. *Surv Ophthalmol* 2001;46(2):117–42.

14. Singh, A. D., Nouri, M., Shields, C. L. et al. Treatment of retinal capillary hemangioma. *Ophthalmology* 2002;109(10):1799–806.

15. Gray, R. H. and Gregor, Z. J. Acquired peripheral retinal telangiectasia after retinal surgery. *Retina* 1994;14(1):10–3.

16. Inoue, M., Yamazaki, K., Shinoda, K. et al. A clinicopathologic case report on macular hole associated with von Hippel-Lindau disease: A novel ultrastructural finding of wormlike, wavy tangles of filaments. *Graefes Arch Clin Exp Ophthalmol* 2004;242(10):881–6.

17. Schwartz, P. L., Fastenberg, D. M. and Shakin, J. L. Management of macular puckers associated with retinal angiomas. *Ophthalmic Surg* 1990;21(8):550–6.

18. Laatikainen, L., Immonen, I. and Summanen, P. Peripheral retinal angiomalike lesion and macular pucker. *Am J Ophthalmol* 1989;108(5):563–6.

19. Ferguson, A. and Singh, J. Total exudative detachment as a first presentation of von Hippel Lindau disease. *Br J Ophthalmol* 2002;86(6):701–2.

20. Loewenstein, J. I. Bilateral macular holes in von Hippel–Lindau disease. *Arch Ophthalmol* 1995;113(2):143–4.

21. Machemer, R. and Williams, J. M. Sr. Pathogenesis and therapy of traction detachment in various retinal vascular diseases. *Am J Ophthalmol* 1988;105(2):170–81.

22. Raju, B., Majji, A. B. and Jalali, S. von Hippel angioma in South Indian subjects – A clinical study. *Retina* 2003;23(5):670–4.

23. Raja, D., Benz, M. S., Murray, T. G. et al. Salvage external beam radiotherapy of retinal capillary hemangiomas secondary to von Hippel–Lindau disease: Visual and anatomic outcomes. *Ophthalmology* 2004;111(1):150–3.

24. Garcia-Arumi, J., Sararols, L. H., Cavero, L. et al. Therapeutic options for capillary papillary hemangiomas. *Ophthalmology* 2000;107(1):48–54.
25. Steel, D. H., Williamson, T. H., Laidlaw, D. A. et al. Extent and location of intraretinal and subretinal fluid as prognostic factors for the outcome of patients with optic disk pit maculopathy. *Retina* 2016;36(1):110–8.
26. Garcia-Arumi, J., Guraya, B. C., Espax, A. B. et al. Optical coherence tomography in optic pit maculopathy managed with vitrectomy-laser-gas. *Graefes Arch Clin Exp Ophthalmol* 2004;242(10):819–26.
27. Lincoff, H. and Kreissig, I. Optical coherence tomography of pneumatic displacement of optic disc pit maculopathy. *Br J Ophthalmol* 1998;82(4):367–72.
28. Dureau, P., Attie-Bitach, T., Salomon, R. et al. Renal coloboma syndrome. *Ophthalmology* 2001;108(10):1912–6.
29. Haik, B. G., Greenstein, S. H., Smith, M. E. et al. Retinal detachment in the morning glory anomaly. *Ophthalmology* 1984;91(12):1638–47.
30. Chang, S., Haik, B. G., Ellsworth, R. M. et al. Treatment of total retinal detachment in morning glory syndrome. *Am J Ophthalmol* 1984;97(5):596–600.
31. Steahly, L. P. Retinochoroidal coloboma: Varieties of clinical presentations. *Ann Ophthalmol* 1990;22(1):9–14.
32. Corcostegui, B., Guell, J. L., Garcia-Arumi, J. Surgical treatment of retinal detachment in the choroidal colobomas. *Retina* 1992;12(3):237–41.
33. Gopal, L., Kini, M. M., Badrinath, S. S. and Sharma, T. Management of retinal detachment with choroidal coloboma. *Ophthalmology* 1991;98(11):1622–7.
34. Gopal, L., Badrinath, S. S., Sharma, T. et al. Pattern of retinal breaks and retinal detachments in eyes with choroidal coloboma. *Ophthalmology* 1995;102(8):1212–7.
35. Abboud, E. B. Retinal detachment surgery in Marfan's syndrome. *Retina* 1998;18(5):405–9.
36. Dotrelova, D., Karel, I. and Clupkova, E. Retinal detachment in Marfan's syndrome: Characteristics and surgical results. *Retina* 1997;17(5):390–6.
37. Hubbard, A. D., Charteris, D. G. and Cooling, R. J. Vitreolensectomy in Marfan's syndrome. *Eye* 1998;12 (Pt 3a):412–6.
38. Bading, G., Hillenkamp, J., Sachs, H. G. et al. Long-term safety and functional outcome of combined pars plana vitrectomy and scleral-fixated sutured posterior chamber lens implantation. *Am J Ophthalmol* 2007;144(3):371–7.
39. Johnston, R. L., Charteris, D. G., Horgan, S. E. and Cooling, R. J. Combined pars plana vitrectomy and sutured posterior chamber implant. *Arch Ophthalmol* 2000;118(7):905–10.
40. Abourizk, N., Ishaq, A. M., Arora, T. et al. Ocular surgery in patients with diabetic nephropathy. *Diabetes Care* 1980;3(4):530–2.
41. Fuchino, Y., Hayashi, H., Kono, T. and Ohshima, K. Long-term follow up of visual acuity in eyes with stage 5 retinopathy of prematurity after closed vitrectomy. *Am J Ophthalmol* 1995;120(3):308–16.
42. Capone, A. Jr. and Trese, M. T. Lens-sparing vitreous surgery for tractional stage 4A retinopathy of prematurity retinal detachments. *Ophthalmology* 2001;108(11):2068–70.
43. Chong, L. P., Machemer, R. and de Juan, E. Vitrectomy for advanced stages of retinopathy of prematurity. *Am J Ophthalmol* 1986;102(6):710–6.
44. Seaber, J. H., Machemer, R., Eliott, D. et al. Long-term visual results of children after initially successful vitrectomy for stage V retinopathy of prematurity. *Ophthalmology* 1995;102(2):199–204.
45. Trese, M. T. and Droste, P. J. Long-term postoperative results of a consecutive series of stages 4 and 5 retinopathy of prematurity. *Ophthalmology* 1998;105(6):992–7.

46. Quinn, G. E., Dobson, V., Barr, C. C. et al. Visual acuity in infants after vitrectomy for severe retinopathy of prematurity. *Ophthalmology* 1991;98(1):5–13.

47. Lakhanpal, R. R., Sun, R. L., Albini, T. A. and Holz, E. R. Anatomical success rate after primary three-port lens-sparing vitrectomy in stage 5 retinopathy of prematurity. *Retina* 2006;26(7):724–8.

48. Cusick, M., Charles, M. K., Agron, E. et al. Anatomical and visual results of vitreoretinal surgery for stage 5 retinopathy of prematurity. *Retina* 2006;26(7):729–35.

49. Terasaki, H. and Hirose, T. Late-onset retinal detachment associated with regressed retinopathy of prematurity. *Jpn J Ophthalmol* 2003;47(5):492–7.

50. Tasman, W. Late complications of retrolental fibroplasia. *Ophthalmology* 1979;86(10):1724–40.

51. Kaiser, R. S., Trese, M. T., Williams, G. A. and Cox, M. S. Jr. Adult retinopathy of prematurity: Outcomes of rhegmatogenous retinal detachments and retinal tears. *Ophthalmology* 2001;108(9):1647–53.

52. Sneed, S. R., Pulido, J. S., Blodi, C. F. et al. Surgical management of late-onset retinal detachments associated with regressed retinopathy of prematurity. *Ophthalmology* 1990;97(2):179–83.

53. Tufail, A., Singh, A. J., Haynes, R. J. et al. Late onset vitreoretinal complications of regressed retinopathy of prematurity. *Br J Ophthalmol* 2004;88(2):243–6.

54. Terson, A. De l'hemorrhagie dans le corp vitre au cours de l'hemorrhagie cerebrale. *Clin Ophthalmol* 1900;6:309–12.

55. van Rens, G. H., Bos, P. J. and van Dalen, J. T. Vitrectomy in two cases of bilateral Terson syndrome. *Doc Ophthalmol* 1983;56(1–2):155–9.

56. Weingeist, T. A., Goldman, E. J., Folk, J. C. et al. Terson's syndrome: Clinicopathologic correlations. *Ophthalmology* 1986;93(11):1435–42.

57. Schultz, P. N., Sobol, W. M. and Weingeist, T. A. Long-term visual outcome in Terson syndrome. *Ophthalmology* 1991;98(12):1814–9.

58. Kuhn, F., Morris, R., Witherspoon, C. D. and Mester, V. Terson syndrome: Results of vitrectomy and the significance of vitreous hemorrhage in patients with subarachnoid hemorrhage. *Ophthalmology* 1998;105(3):472–7.

59. Murjaneh, S., Hale, J. E., Mishra, S. et al. Terson's syndrome: Surgical outcome in relation to entry site pathology. *Br J Ophthalmol* 2006;90(4):512–3.

60. Garweg, J. G. and Koerner, F. Outcome indicators for vitrectomy in Terson syndrome. *Acta Ophthalmol* 2009;87(2):222–6.

61. Rubowitz, A. and Desai, U. Nontraumatic macular holes associated with Terson syndrome. *Retina* 2006;26(2):230–2.

62. Lewis, K., Herbert, E. N. and Williamson, T. H. Severe ocular involvement in disseminated intravascular coagulation complicating meningococcaemia. *Graefes Arch Clin Exp Ophthalmol* 2005;243(10):1069–70.

63. Yanai, D., Weiland, J. D., Mahadevappa, M. et al. Visual performance using a retinal prosthesis in three subjects with retinitis pigmentosa. *Am J Ophthalmol* 2007;143(5):820–7.

64. Roessler, G., Laube, T., Brockmann, C. et al. Implantation and explantation of a wireless epiretinal retina implant device: Observations during the EPIRET3 prospective clinical trial. *Invest Ophthalmol Vis Sci* 2009;50(6):3003–8.

Index

Page numbers followed by f and t indicate figures and tables, respectively.